FEEL NOT FOOD

A Workbook to help you become comfortable *feeling* so you stop emotionally *feeding*.

THERESA PAGANINI

This book is dedicated to my mother.
I am who I am because of you.
I do what I do because of you.
You are my inspiration.
I love you, Mom.

CONTENTS

PROLOGUE

My Story

Did you know that, as of today, there are 1,312 books about emotional eating on Amazon? That's a lot of books on one topic! Between the time I finish writing this book and the time you read it, there will probably be dozens more. So, why read this one? I'm not a doctor; I'm not a psychiatrist; I'm not a registered dietitian or even a counselor. Why read a book from someone who doesn't have a number of fancy letters after their name when there are so many other resources available?

Because I am an emotional eater, just like you.

Because I used to be overweight and unhappy, and despite the fact that I am an emotional eater, I am now a fit, healthy and happy woman.

Because I don't just *academically* understand your struggles as a result of research, studies, and work with various patients. I understand your struggles as only another emotional eater can.

Because I am proof that you can succeed at controlling your urge to eat emotionally, lose weight, feel better about yourself and enjoy life despite being an emotional eater.

Because you have nothing to lose by adding another good resource to your library of support.

Let me introduce myself. Hi, my name is Theresa. I am a health coach that specializes in helping people to make behavioral changes. I have a passion for helping people learn to love themselves and live healthy, fulfilling lives. I want to help people recognize their worth so they can experience the most and best out of their lives. I want to help people build their self-confidence so they feel capable of taking on any challenge despite any fear they may feel. I want to help people look in the mirror with pride, rather than disgust, because they overcame one of their greatest challenges.

I want to help emotional eaters, like me, to go from simply surviving to really living. We can't really enjoy the most out of life when so much of our thinking and attention are on food. We can't really experience true happiness and contentment if we are filled with self-disgust or self-hatred.

I know from my own experience. I am an emotional eater who used to allow food to control me. And every time I did, I was filled with self-disgust. I hated myself for my weakness. I woke up thinking about food and went to bed thinking the same way. What I was going to eat at the next meal was usually uppermost in my mind. If I wasn't eating food, I was usually thinking about it. How can we really get the most out of all the wonders of life if our primary wonder is food? The answer is, we can't.

I think I came out of the womb as an emotional eater; at least that's how it always felt.

Whether I was happy, sad or anything in between, food was always there. As a result, food became my...everything. It was my constant companion, my comfort, my joy, my distraction, my punishment. Food was my remedy for all things good and evil.

As a result, my weight became an issue for me, with the self-confidence problems that go along with it. This, in turn, started my love-hate relationship with food. I absolutely loved everything about food, except that it made me fat. It made me fat because I couldn't seem to control myself around it, and that made me hate food because it was better than hating myself for my seeming lack of control.

Enter the guilt-binge cycle. As a child, I could eat and enjoy food without any guilt, so although I ate too much of the wrong things for the wrong reason, I could enjoy it and not regret it when I was finished. Ah, the joys and ignorance of childhood! Unfortunately, as I got older and realized that it wasn't acceptable, attractive, or endearing to be overweight, I started to look at my eating habits differently—and started to hate who I was. I couldn't control my thoughts and actions surrounding food, so I thought that I must be a very weak-willed individual, someone not worth love or respect. Every time I ate something on my "bad" list, I would feel guilty, beat myself up over it, and then binge to punish myself for being weak—which would cause me to feel guilty, beat myself up and binge again...rinse and repeat. Nothing is as self-defeating, deflating and depressing as the guilt-binge cycle. That cycle would just spiral me down into the depths of despair.

I learned this cycle from my mom. My mother has battled obesity and depression my entire life. She was and still is my greatest hero and friend, and yet she hates herself because she can't see the beautiful person she is to everyone else. My mother has a beautiful soul that just wants to take care of everyone else. And yet, she never places any value on that; her only value is on her weight. Growing up, I listened to the awful things she would say about herself and the way she used food to comfort or to punish herself, and I unknowingly adopted the same behaviors.

Towards the end of middle school, I was so frustrated with myself and food that I decided to give it up altogether and became anorexic. This was triggered by moving from school to school and always struggling to make and keep friends. I figured I just wasn't thin enough or pretty enough to fit in. And it is a hell of a lot easier to avoid binging when you aren't eating at all, so that seemed like a good plan to me! Of course, now that I'm an adult I can see I was simply trading one eating disorder for another, and since my true nature is to be a compulsive overeater, the anorexia only lasted as long as it took for me to get a job at a fast food restaurant. It's amazing how quickly my old habits came back when I was surrounded by french fries, cheeseburgers and fried chicken!

By the time I was 20 years old, I was 45 pounds overweight, which is quite a bit for someone under 5 feet tall. I was also very depressed. Instead of dating, going out dancing, hitting the Florida beaches, and all of the other fun things that kids in their early 20's do, I hid out in my apartment, isolated and alone. I had lost all sense of self-worth; I couldn't see beyond my weight to the person that I was. I hated what I saw in the mirror and didn't think the person staring back at me was worthy of love and acceptance. How could anyone love someone with so little self-control? Someone who couldn't stop themselves from gorging on chocolate, and pizza, and chicken wings? Someone who was so weak they couldn't stick to a weight loss plan for longer than a week or two? Who could love someone so...so...so fat?!

Those were the thoughts that went through my mind on a minute-by-minute basis, and even though I had friends that loved me, I couldn't feel that love because I couldn't accept it. I was filled with so much self-loathing and self-disgust that I didn't think I deserved anyone else's love and acceptance. My mother has spent her whole life feeling alone, even though she has always been one of the most popular and loved women in her network. Similarly, although I had friends and family who loved me, I couldn't feel it because I didn't think I deserved it. Instead, I isolated myself in my apartment and became more and more depressed, which triggered emotional eating, which triggered the self-hatred, which triggered depression, which triggered the emotional eating...see the pattern? Not good.

Luckily, and unknowingly, a good friend of mine was the catalyst for breaking that pattern. Actually, it was nothing more than a picture that changed my life. This picture:

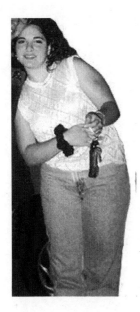

For privacy, I've cut my girlfriend out of the photo, but when she showed me this picture, I literally said, "Great pic! Who's the girl in it with you?" She just looked at me funny and said, "Theresa...that's you." I did a double-take and still didn't recognize myself. I knew I had gained weight since being anorexic and was struggling with depression over my self-image, but there was no way I was that big, was there? I hadn't let my weight get that out of control, had I?

Yes.

Yes, it was me and yes, I had allowed my weight to get that out of control. It was at that point I knew I needed to do something different.

Considering how shocked and horrified I was by that picture, it was obvious that I was living in some sort of denial. And, although seeing that picture shocked me out of that denial and forced me to face the truth about my size, I went into a different form of denial—rationalization. "I don't eat that badly! I exercise! Obviously, I have a thyroid issue and it's not my fault that I'm fat. It's just not fair that everyone else can eat whatever they want, while I eat relatively healthy, and exercise, and I'm so fat!"

If that doesn't make you laugh, this will.

Once I came to the conclusion I had a thyroid issue, I decided I needed to prove it to the doctors so that I could be prescribed a diet pill that would allow me to lose weight. Bariatric surgery and HCG weren't popular yet, so the only solution I could think of was "the diet pill." I admitted to myself that although I ate relatively well and exercised weekly, there was room for improvement. I figured, I'd have to really clean up my diet and exercise more regularly to prove to the doctors that I couldn't lose weight on my own and needed a pill. So, I decided to turn myself into a science experiment. Since the age of 11 I had been studying exercise and nutrition in an attempt to help my mother lose weight, and also stay in control of my own weight. I had studied Exercise and Sports Science in college, and been a personal trainer for many friends at the gym in my past. I knew what to do; I just needed to do it. So, for six months I was going to do everything I had learned from my studies, and no matter what, I wouldn't quit. I figured a doctor would respect a six month attempt at weight loss, whereas they wouldn't respect a one-month attempt. So, even if I didn't lose a pound, I had to keep going. BUT! Only for six months. After that, I was convinced a doctor would realize my plight and prescribe me a diet pill.

Yup, that was my motivation...a diet pill.

So, I did a complete 180° turn and gave up drinking and smoking. I stopped eating out, packed my food each day so I could eat the 5-6 small meals that I knew were recommended, and kept a daily food log to hold myself accountable (and to hand to the doctors at the end of the six months to prove that I, indeed, ate what I should to lose weight). I also started exercising three times per week for 30 minutes (which almost killed me!) and drank a lot of water.

And after 30 days? NOTHING! I didn't lose a single pound—not even an ounce! I'm not joking. At first, I was pissed off because I had worked so hard and I hadn't lost even one pound. How the hell could I go from drinking like a fiend and eating pizza and chicken wings on most nights to a completely healthy lifestyle and not even lose a pound for all of my efforts?! I thought, "Screw this! I'm eating a bacon cheeseburger with fries and a chocolate shake. If I'm going to be fat anyway, I might as well eat whatever I want!" But then I reminded myself that this was an experiment, and that this was actually proving my point, so I just had to stay consistent and keep going, no matter what. I was going to get that damn diet pill if it killed me!

Well, that was enough motivation for me. I kept it up and by the end of month two, my body figured out what was what and I had lost 10 pounds. The rest is history.

So, although my initial motivation to lose weight wasn't really altruistic, it worked. And, I proved to myself that there was physically nothing wrong with me. Like most people on earth, my body will do exactly what I tell it to do. I had simply been speaking the wrong language for too many years.

Also, like most people, I would have gained the weight right back if I hadn't continued using similar eating and exercise patterns like the ones I employed during the weight loss. Isn't that really the hard part? I bet most of you are like me. You get motivated and stay motivated while the weight is coming off, but once we hit our goal, "viola! I'm done!" We think that we are "healed" or "like normal people" just because we hit our goal weight. So we start eating the old foods again; we start slacking off on exercising and rationalize to ourselves about why we don't have the time or energy to do it. Then, the weight starts creeping back up, jeans start feeling tight, and the self-disgust comes roaring back along with the guilt-binge cycle. Then, before you know it, we are back at the same weight—or higher—as when we started. Ugh!

I knew I couldn't let that happen. One of the benefits of growing up with my mother was watching her weight yo-yo as she went on and off diets. Through that, I learned that we can't just stop doing what made us successful in the first place once we reach our goal. This is especially true for emotional eaters, because the moment an emotional eater starts to put weight on again, we beat ourselves up, fall into a depression and then comfort or punish ourselves with food. We have to continue those very same behaviors that made us successful...FOREVER!

So, once I lost the weight, I quickly learned that I needed to figure out how to get a handle on my tendency to emotionally eat if I didn't want to gain the weight back again. That was when I started my real journey, the journey of not only being fit physically, but being fit mentally and emotionally too.

That's the journey I share with you in this book. Every tip, trick and insight come from my own lifelong journey as an emotional eater.

Am I healed? No, I am still an emotional eater, but I now win more battles with food than I lose. Through my journey of transformation, I have learned how to balance self-compassion with accountability so my relationship with food and with myself isn't so negative.

If you are interested in that same transformation, in achieving that same sense of balance and peace with yourself and with food, use this book as a guide on your journey to *Feel Not Food*.

HOW TO USE THIS BOOK

This workbook is meant to help you bring about a transformation. A transformation cannot happen in a day, a week, or even a month. Transformation takes some serious self-reflection, which takes time. I recommend reading the chapters in the order they are written because they build on each other to make the journey easier; however, this is your journey, so if you find it more effective to work chapters in a different order, don't hesitate to do so as each chapter can stand alone.

I also highly recommend re-reading each chapter until you've fully explored everything it has to offer; only you can determine when you have discovered and learned everything each chapter has to contribute to your life. When you begin thinking about these ideas you may find that new thoughts, or new realizations pop up the next day, or every few days, as you come to understand the questions and concepts on a deeper level. One of my clients worked on Chapter 2 for two months before feeling ready to move on to Chapter 3.

This isn't a race but a journey. Take the time you need, and enjoy the process, knowing that having more control of your emotional eating is possible, and can feel empowering.

Emotional eating is probably something you have been battling with for most of your life; you won't be able to overcome it by simply reading a book. The transformation doesn't happen by reading this book; the transformation happens by giving yourself over to the activities in the book without reservations, deadlines, or expectations. If you are willing to open yourself up and face the various truths inside you, you will make great progress on your journey.

I recommend having a separate journal dedicated to your *Feel Not Food* journey in case you need additional space to work on any of the activities in this workbook. Don't let the limited work space in this book stop you from working through an activity in its entirety.

If, at any point, an activity is too difficult to face, simply put the book down and walk away from it until you are ready to continue. Don't skip that activity; the toughest activities are the most vital to your success. However, timing is crucial, so if it isn't the right time to dive that deeply, don't do it, and don't worry about it. Just wait, and continue when you are ready.

If, at any point, an activity brings up some demons that you struggle to deal with, please get some help. Many of us struggle with emotional eating as a result of a trauma from our past. Don't try to cope with the trauma on your own. Please do some research and find a counselor, support group, therapist, psychologist or psychiatrist that can help you work through the trauma so you can finally come to peace with it.

CHAPTER 1

Components of
Long-Term Success

There are a lot of theories about the best way to lose weight and stop emotional eating, and mine is only one of them. This is definitely a topic that has garnered a lot of attention and theories over the years, which is fantastic, because that means we have a lot of resources available to help us. However, finding the right resource is like finding the right spouse. You may go on a number of dates with a variety of people, but that doesn't mean you feel the connection, trust, and camaraderie necessary to commit to a lifelong marriage with them. No, you wait for the right person, and then BAM! That person "gets you" in ways others haven't, and you know they are the one for you. Finding the right weight loss/emotional eating resource is like that, too.

Like me, you may own a variety of books on overcoming emotional eating and/or weight loss, but none of them exactly hit the mark for you. Maybe you didn't like the author's writing style. Or, perhaps a book had too much of a religious or spiritual tone to it, or not enough. Or the message was too blunt and it turned you off, or the opposite, the books was too convoluted and you couldn't make heads or tails out of it. The simple truth is that every single one of those books, videos, support groups and diets help someone, and in many cases a lot of someones. They all work! But do they work for *you*? YOU are the only someone that matters in this case. So, my hope is that you will connect with *my* book, *my* theories, and *my* writing style, so that you will find the support, information and encouragement that you need.

There are various aspects to emotional eating and weight loss. Some are physical, some are psychological, some are spiritual, and some are behavioral. In fact, there is a lot of new information being studied about DNA, the brain, and certain nutrients to help those of us that struggle with food addiction and compulsive eating. And let's be real, if you struggle with emotional eating, there's a good chance you struggle with food addiction and compulsion, as well. So, I highly recommend reading a variety of resources along with my book. This will give you the ability to fight your battle on multiple fronts. I share some good resources on this topic in the back of this book.

With that said, although I recognize there are various physiological and psychological aspects to emotional eating and weight loss, I'm going to focus specifically on the behavioral aspects that you can most easily control, right here and right now.

So, where do we start? Well, until you fully understand what it takes to achieve and maintain success, you can't aim for it. So, let's start with that.

You've probably already experimented with a variety of methods of losing weight quickly, only to gain it back again. Losing weight isn't the hard part; keeping it off is. The reason for that is because ***the weight isn't your problem; it is THE RESULT of your problem.***

Emotional eating is the problem. So, if you only focus on the symptom, then you will rarely experience long-term success. My program is focused on helping you to fix the actual problem of emotional eating so that you can achieve peace, self-confidence and, yes, weight loss.

With that in mind, let's talk about the first component of long-term success.

1. Get the right mindset and set realistic expectations for this journey.

This journey to mental and physical health and weight loss has no destination; it has no end. That is important to understand. Think about it. What has happened every time you have experienced success with a diet or weight loss program? That's right, you hit your goal, thought you were done, and almost immediately started to regain the weight as your old habits crept back in.

The truth is that you may always be an emotional eater. That doesn't mean you will always emotionally eat, that simply means that your initial, knee-jerk reaction to stress, boredom, or strong emotions *may be* to eat. A smaller and healthier body doesn't make that go away. So, coming to accept the fact that this is a never-ending journey is important for your long-term success.

That may seem really depressing and daunting to some of you, but here is the reality: everyone has something in their life that challenges them over and over again throughout their life. Emotional eating is *your* challenge. Your neighbor may be battling clinical depression, your co-worker drug addiction, or your kid's teacher may have obsessive compulsive disorder, etc. Everyone has something that challenges them. Just because you can't see it or don't know about it doesn't mean it doesn't exist. The good news is that although your journey has no destination, it becomes a lot easier with practice and time. The desire to eat when you feel emotions becomes significantly less, and your new habits become so ingrained that actually giving in to the emotional urge to eat becomes the exception rather than the rule. If you think about how rarely you currently win that battle with emotional eating, you can really appreciate how great that news is!

So, if this is a never-ending journey, we've got to pick a journey we can follow for the long haul, which is exactly why fad diets won't work for you. Extreme diets are meant to tackle the symptom of being overweight, not the "illness" of being an emotional eater. Extreme diets are meant to be used only in the short-term and have an end date. You, on the other hand, need something you can do for life. So, no more fad dieting...deal?

So, if we aren't going to diet, what are we going to do?

2. We are going to eat with the intention of improving our health and maximizing our nutrition, not focus on losing weight.

Dieting is all about what you **can't** eat in order to lose weight. Instead, I want you to focus on what you **should** eat for maximum nutrition and enjoyment. When we think in terms of what we "can" and "can't" eat, foods become "good" or "bad." Labeling food as either good or bad gives it a lot of power over you. Eating "good" foods then has the power to make you feel proud, slim, powerful, and in control. Eating "bad" foods has the power to make you feel guilt, shame, self-disgust, and fat. Food doesn't deserve to have that power. It doesn't ask for that power. So, let's not give it that power.

Instead, let's look at food simply as the language we use to speak to our body. How we talk to our body determines how our body will respond. **_When we talk to our bodies with love and respect, we will get love and respect back. When we speak with hatred or disregard, our bodies respond in kind._** Speaking with love means giving your body the nutrition it needs to look and feel its best. This isn't the same for everyone, so like learning any new language, it will take practice to get it right. Some bodies require more protein, others more fat, and others more carbohydrates. It is important to understand what makes your body feel it's most energetic and competent so you can experience and enjoy your life to its fullest.

Did you notice that I mentioned the importance of enjoying your food and your life? That's another component of long-term success.

3.   Enjoy your food!

The whole reason why it's so hard to stay on a diet is because it's boring, restrictive, or tasteless! Whenever people talk about eating healthy, they usually use salads, or grilled chicken, steamed vegetables and brown rice as examples. Although those are definitely healthy foods that will help you lose weight, they can become tasteless and boring over time! You can't live the rest of your life that way; it's just not realistic. Why do we feel as if we are only doing well when we are suffering? I don't get it. If I am going to eat healthy for the rest of my life, I'm going to make sure that it's delicious! My philosophy is simple. I want to enjoy life. I can't live without food. Therefore, to enjoy life I must enjoy food. Not a bad philosophy, right? ☺ The key is learning how to make the nutritious delicious and the delicious nutritious. I still eat hamburgers, pizza, tacos, and desserts; I just cook and eat them differently. I cook and eat food with the intent of speaking the language of love and respect to my body through nutrition.

This brings up the next component of long-term success:

4.   Eat mindfully.

If we are going to eat with the intention of speaking a love language to our bodies, then we need to be aware of what we are saying. Besides, how can you truly enjoy your food if you have no idea you are even eating it? Unfortunately, many of us eat unconsciously.

Have you ever polished off a bag or a plate of _**fill in the blank**_, and didn't even realize what you were doing until you were done? That's the height of unconscious eating. We need to change that. We should be aware of everything we put in our mouths, and not only aware but mindful. If our goal is to enjoy food as well as use it as a love language to our body, then we need to pay attention to it.

Going forward, make a conscious decision to eat or not to eat EVERYTHING you put in your mouth, whether it is a carrot stick or a brownie. Before you put anything in your mouth, think about what you are doing and why, then make the decision of whether you really want to eat it or not. Once that mindful decision is made, whether it is to eat a carrot or a brownie, ENJOY IT!

When was the last time a person in the health and weight loss industry told you to enjoy your brownie? Well, if it is a mindful decision, I encourage it! And that's the fifth component of long-term success:

5. Break the link between negative emotions and food.

There are two ways in which we link negative emotions and food. One, we view food as the enemy and categorize certain foods as "bad." Once we categorize a food as bad, it immediately triggers negative emotions when we eat it. Emotions such as guilt, self-disgust, and shame are destructive emotions that tend to cause binges, which bring on even stronger destructive emotions, which cause further binging, etc. However, once a brownie simply becomes a brownie again, we no longer associate it with guilt, self-disgust or shame and can actually enjoy it and move on with our lives.

The other way we link negative emotions with food is by using food for comfort and/or as a distraction when we are upset. The last thing we should do when we are upset is eat, simply because, as emotional eaters, we are incapable of being mindful about eating when we are emotional. To break the link between negative emotions and food we need to become more comfortable feeling "negative" emotions and working through them appropriately, and find new ways of finding comfort when we need it.

This leads us to component number six:

6. Allow yourself to experience all emotions, both "positive" and "negative."

Emotional eating is a result of avoiding emotions that we don't want to feel.

There are no "negative" emotions; there are simply negative reactions to emotions. Anger, sadness, frustration, rejection, fear and loneliness are only a few of the emotions that are often labeled as "negative" or "bad." These are not negative at all! These are character-building emotions.

Think about the people you most admire and respect. Now ask yourself, "what hardships have these people overcome?" I'll bet you a million dollars that you are able to name various hardships or obstacles that those people overcame.

Challenges make us smarter, stronger and more resilient. Hardships, challenges, strife—or whatever you want to call it— produce strong emotions, which means that the people you admire have experienced "negative" emotions, dealt with them, and then overcame them. That's what has built their character. That is why you admire and respect them.

If you are suffering from low self-confidence, is it easier for you to understand why you don't admire or respect yourself? If you avoid feeling emotions when you're going through the tough stuff, you stop learning, growing, and strengthening your character. You live in fear and hide away instead. It's time to stop being afraid and start fully living your life, both the good and the bad, without needing food for comfort.

Not needing food for comfort—this is a very important topic, so there is an entire chapter dedicated to it later in the book. For now, let's take this theme and take it a step farther.

Just as we have been taking the power away from our emotions, we've been giving unnecessary power to food. Component number 7 for success is:

7. Stop giving food responsibilities it doesn't deserve.

Food is just food; Eating food is just a way to nourish our bodies so we can enjoy our life, be healthy and feel our best. Food is not a reward, nor is it a healthy way to comfort ourselves. Food shouldn't be the center of attention at our parties, and it doesn't have to be the foundation of every date we go on. Eating food doesn't have to be our only way of celebrating, and it shouldn't be the way we distract ourselves from something we don't want to deal with. If food has become any of these things to us it is only because we have given it that role. For our short-term and long-term success at overcoming our emotional eating, and to help us lose weight, we need to find some new:

- Reward systems
- Activities to do outside of the home
- Ways to socialize and entertain
- Ways to comfort
- Ways to celebrate
- Ways to distract
- Ways to deal with stress

It's not surprising, considering how crazy, busy, and stressful all of our lives have become, that more and more people are becoming emotional eaters as a way to deal with their stress.

This brings us to the next component of long-term success:

8. Find ways to reduce the amount of stress in your life. Then, find more effective ways to handle the stress you can't avoid.

Notice that the first course of action is to *remove* stress. Most of us try to find ways to deal with all of the stress in our lives instead of getting rid of it. The world has become a crazy place of constant action. We are all trying to fit more into our 24-hour day than ever before. As a result, everything that is really important to us starts to suffer. We don't have time to take care of ourselves; we don't have enough time with our family and friends; we don't have enough time to stop, to be aware of our thoughts and feelings or to make sense of our emotions. We don't have time to stop and actually enjoy the lives we've created. We don't have enough time to get a good night's sleep; we don't have time be creative or dream. We simply don't have time.

Not having enough time for all these important things is what causes the ultimate stress in our lives. By limiting our opportunities to think, feel, and connect with other people or ourselves we feel this constant sense of dissatisfaction and emptiness that we try to fill with other things—like "stuff," responsibilities, or activities. It is almost manic. We feel this compulsion to own more, do more, be more, and yet none of it truly fulfills us.

It is time to choose what you want out of life, to figure out what is really important to you, and then start getting rid of the rest. Look at all of the responsibilities that you have in your life. Are they fulfilling? Is the satisfaction and fulfillment you get from those responsibilities worth the time and effort you dedicate to them? If not, let go of them. How about all of your "stuff?" Do you own it, or does it own you? What "stuff" aren't you using, enjoying, and benefiting from? What "stuff" do you have that is so expensive that you spend more time working to pay for it than you do using and enjoying it? Get rid of it!

By prioritizing what is important to you and creating a life that matches your priorities, you will significantly reduce your stress. This will give you time to stop, breathe, relax, and enjoy your life. Doesn't that sound nice? Who needs to eat emotionally, or for comfort, when you feel relaxed and are enjoying life? Exactly!

Unfortunately, another cause of stress in our life is people. It isn't as easy to get rid of people as it is to get rid of "stuff." But, and this is a really big but, (not *your* butt! ☺), it is really important to your success to surround yourself with people who will support you on your journey. Studies have proven that long-term success using any weight loss system is heavily dependent on having a strong support system—which takes us to component number nine.

9. Create a strong support system you can count on when the going gets tough.

Who will encourage you to make a healthier choice at a restaurant, or in a social setting? Who will cheer you on when you lose your motivation and want to quit? Who will pick you up, brush you off, give you a hug, and push you in the right direction when you get off track on your journey away from emotional eating? Those are the people that you need to talk with about your journey. Those are the people that you need to ask for help. Those are the people that you need to be willing to be vulnerable with and to trust—because they will have your back, even when you don't.

Once you know who you need in your support system, you need to define exactly what support you want each of them to give you. Support is a finicky thing. We all have our own definition of what support is, and it's important that you know what your version of it is before you ask others to support you. Tell them what support means to you, and what you need from them. That sets them up for success, so they can help you the way you need it. You don't want them to give you *their* version of support. So, help them to help you by clearly outlining what you need from them.

I make all of that sound really simple. And in truth, it IS simple; what it isn't is easy.

As I mentioned earlier, the journey to health is never-ending. It will have ups and downs, detours and roadblocks—and that's normal! Being perfect is not only unrealistic, it isn't even an option. So, please let go of any idea of being perfect. Trying to be perfect also adds stress, and you don't need that. I have outlined nine components of success so far, and you are going to have moments of success and failure with each of them. It's ok. Accept that.

This brings us to the final component.

10. Self-acceptance. You are not now, nor will you ever be, perfect. And that's ok.

In fact, you are perfectly imperfect, like every other person on Earth. That really put-together mom at your kid's school, the one who always looks perfect, is always in a good mood, and has well-behaved kids is as imperfect as you are—but in different ways. That successful co-worker who continues to get promoted and receives awards for outstanding performance is as imperfect as you are—but in different ways. Stop comparing yourself to other people. It does you no good because you don't know their whole story. You don't know what their insecurities are, you don't know what their challenges are, and you don't know what their shortcomings are. You don't know them. You see only what they allow you to see, and very few people put their insecurities and weaknesses on display for everyone to see. If you are overweight, unfortunately, your struggle is harder to hide so you feel vulnerable and exposed. That feeds your insecurity. But the truth is, having extra weight can be fixed. That "perfect" mom or co-worker may be dealing with something much worse that is easier to hide but impossible to "fix". Don't let your insecurities and assumptions mislead you into thinking that someone else has it better than you.

Self-acceptance means loving yourself, even if there are things about you or your life you'd like to change. If you can learn to appreciate your value to the world, exactly as you are today, you will immediately begin experiencing the world in a whole new light. You'll feel things you've never felt before. You'll do things you've never done before. You'll say things you've never said before. You'll see things you've never seen before.

The simple truth is that you are more than your weight. By allowing your weight or your illness of emotional eating to define who you are, you are taking away your ability to fully experience and enjoy your life, and your ability to truly connect with other people. You are taking away your ability to feel love and acceptance from others. You are taking away your ability to show the world who you really are. You are taking away your confidence that you can contribute to the world around you. It doesn't have to be like this, and you deserve all those experiences.

It's time to stop cheating yourself—and the world around you! It's time to experience the wonder of who you really are. When you can finally accept everything about yourself, and accept you are imperfect (like all the rest of us), you'll start to experience life more fully, and to realize everything it has to offer—and everything YOU have to offer.

CHAPTER SUMMARY

10 components of overcoming emotional eating and helping you to lose weight, for both short-term and long-term success:

1. Get the right mindset and set realistic expectations for your journey.
2. Eat for health and nutrition, not weight loss.
3. Enjoy your food!
4. Eat mindfully.
5. Break the link between "negative" emotions and food.
6. Allow yourself to feel all emotions, both "negative" and "positive."
7. Stop giving food an importance and power it doesn't deserve.
8. Reduce the stress in your life, and find healthier, more effective ways of dealing with the stress that can't be removed.
9. Create a strong support system you can count on when the going gets tough.

10. Accept that you are not, nor will you ever be, perfect—just like all of us!

Now that we know where we want to go, let's take a closer look at where we currently are.

CHAPTER 2

Evaluation

Let the journey begin! As I mentioned in Chapter 1, although there are many variables that impact emotional eating, we are going to focus solely on our behaviors, and specifically the 10 behaviors I outlined in Chapter 1. Those 10 behaviors will help you to achieve long-term success in overcoming your emotional eating. However, if you try to tackle all 10 behaviors at once, you are going to get overwhelmed and quit.

Instead, let's figure out which behaviors you are already strong at and which you could use some improvement on. Self-awareness is extremely important on this journey; unless you are aware of what you are thinking, saying and doing, you can't keep yourself accountable for consistently performing these new, healthier, happier behaviors.

So, step one of this journey is figuring out where you currently stand. To help you figure that out, I've created an evaluation for each behavior. Based on how you score, you will know which behaviors to focus on first as you begin to transform your thoughts, self-talk, and actions.

Be completely honest on these evaluations. Some of you may want to score yourself higher so you don't look so bad. Some of you will want to score yourselves lower just to prove how bad you are. No one else will see your scores, and neither of those approaches will help you. Remember, there is no good or bad, it is just what is. So, let's see what is!

For each question, circle the number on the spectrum that best describes your current state. 0 means you aren't doing, thinking, or feeling it at all and 10 means you do it consistently, all of the time.

GETTING THE RIGHT MINDSET

1. I am excited to change my focus from weight loss to overcoming the root problem of emotional eating.

    0   1   2   3   4   (5)   6   7   8   9   10

2. I resent the fact that I will have to eat healthy and exercise consistently for the rest of my life if I want to achieve and maintain my ideal weight.

    0   1   2   3   4   5   6   7   (8)   9   10

3. I am excited to learn new, long-term lifestyle habits instead of doing another fad diet.

    0   1   2   3   4   5   (6)   7   8   9   10

4. I worry that I will lose my motivation on this journey if the weight loss does not happen quickly.

    0   1   2   3   4   5   6   7   8   (9)   10

5. I accept the fact that this is a life-long journey and that hitting my goal weight does not mean I am "cured" of emotional eating.

    0   1   2   3   4   5   6   7   (8)   9   10

6. I feel nervous about digging deep and possibly unearthing some demons I'm not ready to face.

    0   1   (2)   3   4   5   6   7   8   9   10

Scoring

Add your scores from statements 1, 3, and 5, and write it down. Now add your scores from statements 2, 4, and 6, and write it down. Subtract the second total from the first.

Score: _____

If your final score is greater than 5, you are strong at this behavior and have the right mindset for this journey.

EATING FOR HEALTH AND NUTRITION RATHER THAN WEIGHT LOSS

1. I am willing to take the power away from food and stop considering foods as either good or bad.

   0   1   2   3   4   5   6   7   8   (9)   10

2. Instead of eating what I have always eaten, I am willing to start reviewing all of my options and choosing the food that will best nourish my body.

   0   1   2   3   4   5   6   7   (8)   9   10

3. I am nervous to focus on nutrition rather than weight loss; I fear I will continue to gain weight if I don't count calories or put myself on a strict diet.

   0   1   2   3   4   5   6   7   8   (9)   10

4. I like the idea of using food as a language of love to my body.

   0   1   2   3   4   5   6   7   (8)   9   10

5. I am willing to ignore the media and my well-intentioned friends and family, and instead pay attention to my body in order to determine what percentage of fats, proteins, and carbohydrates make my body look and feel its best.

   0   1   2   3   4   5   6   7   8   (9)   10

6. I am willing to try new foods and cooking methods in order to expand my palate and increase my nutrition.

   0   1   2   3   4   5   6   7   (8)   9   10

Scoring

Add together the score for each statement.

Score: ___51___

<20 = needs attention
20-34 = average
>35 = strong

ENJOYING YOUR FOOD AND YOUR LIFE

1. I am willing to change my self-dialogue so that I can enjoy healthy and nutritious food that also tastes delicious without feeling guilty.

    0   1   2   3   4   5   (6)   7   8   9   10

2. I am nervous/concerned about the amount of time and work it will take to be healthy.

    0   1   2   3   4   5   6   7   (8)   9   10

3. I am willing to spend time each week researching healthier recipes for my favorite meals, so I can enjoy my food while nourishing my body.

    0   1   2   3   4   5   6   7   (8)   9   10

4. I am willing to proactively look up nutrition information on restaurant food before going out, in order to make the healthiest and most satisfying choice.

    0   1   2   3   4   5   6   (7)   8   9   10

5. I will not feel guilty for ordering a nutritious item at a restaurant just because it is not the lowest calorie item on the menu.

    0   1   2   3   4   5   6   7   (8)   9   10

6. I like the idea of allowing all of my senses to enjoy my meal before I begin eating it. I will notice and appreciate the various colors, scents, and textures in my meal in order to better enjoy it.

    0   1   2   3   4   5   6   7   8   (9)   10

Scoring

Add together the score for each statement.

Score: ___46___

<20 = needs attention
20-34 = average
>35 = strong

EATING MINDFULLY

1. For the next 2 weeks, I am willing to stop for a full 30 seconds before eating or drinking **ANYTHING** to ensure I am eating/drinking mindfully as well as confident my choice is both nutritious and delicious.

   0   1   2   3   4   5   6   7   (8)   9   10

2. I am willing to immediately stop and assess both my hunger and my choices if I become aware in the midst of unconsciously eating.

   0   1   2   3   4   5   (6)   7   8   9   10

3. I am willing to let go of guilt if I make a mindful decision to eat something more delicious than nutritious.

   0   1   2   3   4   5   6   7   (8)   9   10

4. For the next 2 weeks I am willing to measure my food in order to learn proper portion sizes, which will help me eat more mindfully.

   0   1   2   3   4   5   6   7   (8)   9   10

Scoring:

Add together the score for each statement.

Score: ___30___

<12 = needs attention
12-20 = average
>20 = strong

BREAKING THE LINK BETWEEN NEGATIVE EMOTIONS AND FOOD

1. I am willing to eat delicious foods without guilt as long as I eat them mindfully.

   0   1   2   3   4   5   6   7   (8)   9   10

2. I am willing to adopt positive self-talk during those times I eat foods that are more delicious than nutritious.

   0   1   2   3   4   5   6   7   (8)   9   10

3. I'm worried I'll feel like a fraud when I change my self-dialogue from negative to positive.

   0   1   2   3   (4)   5   6   7   8   9   10

4. For the next 2 weeks, I am willing to avoid eating **ANYTHING** when I feel a strong emotion that disturbs my peace of mind.

   0   1   2   3   4   5   (6)   7   8   9   10

Scoring:

Add the score for statements 1, 2, and 4 then subtract the score from statement 3.

Score: ___26___

<12 = needs attention
12-20 = average
>20 = strong

EXPERIENCING ALL EMOTIONS, BOTH GOOD AND BAD

1. Feeling and experiencing certain emotions scares me.

    0   1   2   3   4   5   6   7   (8)   9   10

2. I am nervous to identify which emotions cause me to overeat and explore what it is about those emotions that scare me.

    0   1   2   3   4   5   (6)   7   8   9   10

3. I am willing to explore the necessity of feeling sadness, anger, frustration, hurt, etc in order to live a happier, more fulfilled life.

    0   1   2   3   4   5   6   7   8   (9)   10

4. I am willing to learn how to face all of my emotions head on without the use of food.

    0   1   2   3   4   5   6   7   (8)   9   10

5. I am afraid of losing control if I allow myself to feel "negative" emotions.

    0   1   2   3   4   (5)   6   7   8   9   10

Scoring:

Add the scores for statements 1, 2, and 5.

Score: _____19_____

>12 = needs attention
8-12 = average
0-7 = strong

Add the scores for statements 3 and 4.

Score: _____17_____

<10 = needs attention
10-14 = average
15-20 = strong

STOP GIVING FOOD RESPONSIBILITIES IT DOESN'T DESERVE

I am willing to look for and practice alternative methods for
_____ without using food:

1. Celebrating

    0   1   2   3   4   5   6   (7)   8   9   10

2. Socializing

    0   1   2   3   4   (5)   6   7   8   9   10

3. Rewarding

    0   1   2   3   4   5   6   7   8   (9)   10

4. Comforting

    0   1   2   3   4   5   6   7   8   (9)   10

5. Distracting

    0   1   2   3   4   5   6   7   8   (9)   10

6. Dealing with Stress

    0   1   2   3   4   5   6   7   (8)   9   10

7. Dealing with Boredom

    0   1   2   3   4   5   6   (7)   8   9   10

Scoring

Add together the score for each statement.

Score: _____54_____

<21 = needs attention
21-42 = average
>42 = strong

REDUCE THE AMOUNT OF STRESS IN YOUR LIFE

1. I am willing to unemotionally evaluate the different stressors in my life.

   0   1   2   3   4   (5)   6   7   8   9   10

2. I am willing to actively reduce my stress in order to make my health a higher priority.

   0   1   2   3   4   5   6   7   (8)   9   10

I believe taking care of me is more important than:

3. Working overtime

   0   1   2   3   4   5   6   7   8   (9)   10

4. Household chores

   0   1   2   3   4   5   6   7   8   (9)   10

5. Socializing

   0   1   2   3   4   5   (6)   7   8   9   10

6. Taking on my friend's responsibilities

   0   1   2   3   4   5   6   7   8   (9)   10

7. Taking on my family's responsibilities

   0   1   2   3   4   5   (6)   7   8   9   10

8. Taking care of my "stuff" (ex: house, yard, car, etc)

   0   1   2   3   4   5   6   7   (8)   9   10

Scoring

Add together the score for each statement.

Score: ___60___

<24 = needs attention
24-48 = average
>48 = strong

CREATE A STRONG SUPPORT SYSTEM YOU CAN COUNT ON WHEN THE GOING GETS TOUGH

1. I know who will support me best on my emotional eating/weight loss journey.

   0   1   (2)   3   4   5   6   7   8   9   10

2. I can easily define what type of support I want from each person in my support system.

   0   1   (2)   3   4   5   6   7   8   9   10

3. I am willing to ask for help when I need it.

   0   1   2   (3)   4   5   6   7   8   9   10

4. I am willing to receive help even when I don't ask for it because I know my support team has my best interests at heart.

   0   1   2   3   (4)   5   6   7   8   9   10

5. I am comfortable communicating my needs to the people in my support system.

   0   1   (2)   3   4   5   6   7   8   9   10

If you have children...

6. I am willing to ask for support from my children.

   0   1   2   3   (4)   5   6   7   8   9   10

7. I am willing to hold my children accountable for supporting me through this journey.

   0   1   2   3   (4)   5   6   7   8   9   10

Scoring

Add together the scores for each of the statements.

Score: _____ 21 _____

If you only answered questions 1-5, then:

<15 = needs attention
16-30 = average
>30 = strong

If you answered questions 1-7, then:

<21 = needs attention
21-42 = average
>42 = strong

ACCEPT THAT YOU ARE NOT, NOR WILL YOU EVER BE PERFECT

1. I expect me to be perfect.

   0   1   2   3   (4)   5   6   7   8   9   10

2. I expect others to be perfect.

   0   1   2   3   (4)   5   6   7   8   9   10

3. I berate myself for making mistakes.

   0   1   (2)   3   4   5   6   7   8   9   10

4. I have little patience for my mistakes, big or small.

   0   1   2   3   4   (5)   6   7   8   9   10

5. I am willing to demonstrate self-compassion when I make mistakes.

   0   1   2   3   4   (5)   6   7   8   9   10

6. I dislike learning new things if I don't catch onto them quickly; they make me feel stupid.

   0   1   2   3   4   5   6   7   (8)   9   10

7. I hate my body.

   0   1   2   3   4   5   (6)   7   8   9   10

8. I am willing to learn to love and/or accept my body in its imperfection.

   0   1   2   3   4   5   6   7   (8)   9   10

9. I am afraid that if I learn to love my body as it is I will lose my motivation to lose weight.

   0   1   2   3   4   5   6   7   8   (9)   10

10. I often feel judged by others.

0   1   2   3   4   5   6   7   8   (9)   10

11. I understand that I am in control of my reactions and emotions; other people cannot make me feel inferior unless I let them.

0   1   2   3   4   5   (6)   7   8   9   10

Scoring

Add together the score for each of the statements.

Score: ___66___

>65 = needs attention, 50-64 = average, <49 = strong

Whew! I wonder how many of you would have bought this book if you knew you had to take 10 evaluations in one of the very first chapters ☺. Luckily, these aren't pass or fail evaluations!! They are, however, very reflective and revealing evaluations, so I'd like for you to walk away from the book for a day or two, then come back and look over your answers to see if you agree with the numbers you chose. You may find that your answers change after some reflection. Once you are confident you've accurately evaluated yourself, you can move onto chapter 3.

In Chapter 3, we will discuss what to do with these results...

CHAPTER 3

Making Positive Changes to Your Behaviors

This is only Chapter 3 and you've already experienced your first success! You've honestly evaluated where you currently stand regarding the 10 behaviors. Now, you can easily see what changes you need to make to achieve success! Unfortunately, change is that little constant in life that causes us varying degrees of anxiety and stress. Some of us handle change better than others, but change tends to cause some level of discomfort to all of us.

You purchased this book because you recognize that you need to make changes to your mind, body and spirit in order to overcome your emotional eating and/or weight loss challenges.

Recognizing that you need to make changes?
That's relatively easy.

Wanting the results of those changes?
That's VERY easy.

Actually making the changes and sticking with them?
That's hard!

The goal of this chapter is to help you identify what changes you need to make, based on your evaluation scores from the last chapter, and to honestly evaluate your willingness to adopt them.

After completing the evaluations in the last chapter, you should have a clearer idea of which of the 10 behaviors will require you to make the most changes. You may feel overwhelmed by how much you need to change to be successful, long-term. The good news is that any and all changes will have a positive impact on your success. You don't have to tackle everything all at once to experience success. In fact, if you try to tackle everything at once you are more likely to fail.

Emotional eaters tend to live in a black and white world filled with "all or nothing" moments. You either work like a dervish or laze around all day. You are either really happy with life or completely depressed. You are either on a really restrictive diet or binge eating. You are either a social butterfly or a recluse. Does any of this sound familiar? Living life in these extremes is exhausting. In fact, living in these extremes guarantees failure, which is why we can't maintain the "high;" it isn't realistic. Neither is attacking this journey with an "all or nothing" mentality. So, let's set a ground rule that you will resist the all or nothing mentality and practice living "in the gray" from now on. There's a lot of space between all and nothing (black or white), so let's spend more time exploring that gray area.

The first way in which you can do that is by taking a look at your evaluation results and determining the best place to start your journey. In a black and white world, we would try to conquer all of our weaknesses at once and try to change everything. Guaranteed failure! So, in our new, beautiful, gray world we are going to be more strategic and set ourselves up for success.

> Extremes are exhausting. Let's break that "black and white" thinking and practice thinking and living in "the gray."

Let's start by reviewing the evaluation results from the previous chapter and identifying which of the 10 behaviors will be the easiest for us to adopt and which will be the hardest. List the 10 behaviors below in order of easiest to hardest, based on your scoring.

1. _____

2. _____

3. _____

4. _____

5. _____

6. _____

7. _____

8. _____

9. _____

10. _____

Now that you've determined which behaviors will be easiest and hardest to change, let's focus on numbers 1 and 2. On any long-term journey, it is important you experience success early and often, otherwise you'll lose your motivation. You will see and experience success more easily by focusing on the behaviors that are the easiest to change. So, despite your instincts, which may be to start

> You will not experience different results if you keep doing the same thing. So, fight your instincts, trust mine, and start your journey focusing on behaviors 1 and 2 on your list.

with the bottom three behaviors on your list, I want you to trust me and start with the top two.

Looking at the first behavior you listed above, I want you to describe what this behavior would be like if you were to adopt it and make it part of your life.

For example, let's say "Enjoy your food" is number 1 on my list. This would be my description of what this behavior would be like if I were to make it part of my life:

1. Find healthy recipes for my favorite foods like pizza, burgers, Thai green curry, fried rice, ice cream, cookies, etc.
2. Look for healthy options that I can order at my favorite restaurants that are both delicious and nutritious.
3. Stop for 30 seconds before eating each meal and involve all of my senses so I can fully enjoy the meal on every level.
4. Stop multitasking while I eat. No more watching television, working, playing on my phone, or playing video games while I eat. I need to pay attention to and enjoy my food.
5. Eat slower. Take smaller bites, chew each bite more thoroughly, and pause throughout my meal to truly enjoy my meal and be aware of when I feel full.
6. Experiment with spices to add more flavor to my dishes.
7. Experiment with textures to determine what gives me that pleasant mouth feel I enjoy with foods that are more delicious than nutritious.

Once again, this is just an example. I want you to complete this same activity, using my example as a guide, but doing it with *your* number 1 behavior.

This list should give you a clear idea of what it will take to succeed at adopting the overall behavior. I'm going to call the items in your list your "sub-behaviors," the various actions you will need to take to succeed at the overall behavior change you want to make. Looking over your list, I bet there are some sub-behaviors that you are excited about and others that make you sigh heavily with resignation.

If we go back to my sample list, I would get excited about finding new recipes for my favorite foods, but I would not be excited about putting away my phone while I eat. I usually eat alone. What the heck am I going to do to entertain myself, by myself, while I'm eating?! Although the obvious answer is to enjoy the meal, that may not excite me enough to turn off my phone. As I mentioned earlier, there is a big difference between *wanting* results and *being willing* to change to get those results. It is very easy to *want*; it isn't nearly as easy to *do*. So, the question I would ask myself is, "Although I'm not excited about putting away my phone, am I willing to do it to achieve the results I want?"

That is the very question I want you to ask yourself about each of the sub-behaviors you listed above. Are you willing to consistently do that sub-behavior to achieve the results you want?

This question isn't meant to guilt you into complying. You've spent enough of your life driven by guilt. Guilt is a big driver in a black and white world. But, we are now living in a gray world where we have lots of options in between all and nothing. So, this question is simply meant to raise your self-awareness and make you think honestly about what you are and are not willing to do RIGHT NOW on this journey. Just because you aren't willing to do the sub-behavior as you wrote it doesn't mean there isn't another way to do it.

I have quite a few clients that refuse to eat breakfast in the morning. They know it's good for them, but they feel nauseous at the thought of eating so early in the morning, or they don't have time to make breakfast, or they have no desire to make it, or they simply don't want to eat first thing in the morning. Okay, fine then, no eating breakfast—for now. But then I always ask them if they are willing to *drink* their breakfast. It's fast, easy, delicious, nutritious and easier to swallow first thing in the morning than food. The answer is almost always "yes!" Just because they weren't willing to adopt the *healthiest* behavior didn't mean they weren't willing to adopt a *healthier* behavior. The same goes for you and your list of sub-behaviors. Just because you aren't willing to do a sub-behavior the way you listed it doesn't mean you should give up on it entirely. You simply come up with an alternate solution. Isn't living in a gray world wonderful!?!?

So, with all of this in mind, I want you to go back to your list of sub-behaviors. Place a **+** sign next to each one that you are willing to adopt, as is. Put a **Δ** next to the sub-behaviors you aren't yet ready to adopt the way you wrote them.

Now, let's go play in the gray. For every sub-behavior with a delta sign (**Δ**), I want you to do some soul searching and figure out why you are unwilling to adopt it. Then, use that information and play in the gray, and modify the behavior until it is something you *are* willing to adopt.

Sub-Behavior:

Why I'm Unwilling to Adopt It:

Play in the Gray:

Sub-Behavior:

Why I'm Unwilling to Adopt It:

Play in the Gray:

Sub-Behavior:

Why I'm Unwilling to Adopt It:

Play in the Gray:

Sub-Behavior:

Why I'm Unwilling to Adopt It:

Play in the Gray:

(If you need more space to work on this activity, continue working on this in your dedicated Feel Not Food journal.)

How are you feeling, so far? Excited that things are becoming clearer? Successful, because you are creating a realistic strategy to beat your tendencies to eat emotionally? Relief, since you don't have to be perfect, just better? Capable, because you get to choose the changes that you are willing to make?

Take a second and evaluate how you are feeling. Don't censor yourself, don't hide, don't push your emotions down—FEEL! A huge part of this journey is becoming more in tune with your emotions and allowing yourself to feel them. Take a moment and write about how you are feeling at this point in the process (it may not be all unicorns and rainbows) and continue in your journal if you need additional space.

The goal is improvement,
NOT PERFECTION!

Okay, back to the journey!

Now that you know what you are willing to do to succeed, the final step is to determine *when* you are willing to start. Are you ready to start implementing these sub-behaviors today? If not, when? Remember, you are now living in the gray, so there is no expectation that you have to adopt all of these sub-behaviors successfully 100% of the time. The goal is improvement, not perfection. So, let me ask you again—when are you ready to start practicing these sub-behaviors? Today? Tomorrow? Next Monday?

Pick a date and write it here: _____

Now reflect on why you chose that date. We are taking emotion out of your interaction with food, so I want this to be a logical, well thought out decision, not an impulse.

Why I chose this date to begin using my new sub-behaviors:

Now that you've had time to reflect on the date you chose, are you satisfied you made the right decision? If not, then change the date you put down to one that makes more sense for you.

Okay, good!

It's time to go through these same steps for the second behavior you are going to tackle. Use the spaces below to work through each step in the willingness process to set you up for success.

List the sub-behaviors that best describe what your number 2 behavior looks like for you.

Place a **+** sign next to each one that you are willing to adopt as you wrote it. Put a **Δ** next to the sub-behaviors you aren't yet ready to adopt the way you wrote about them.

Now, go play in the gray. For every sub-behavior with a delta, I want you to modify the behavior until it is something you *are* willing to adopt.

Sub-Behavior:
Why I'm Unwilling to Adopt It:
Play in the Gray:

Sub-Behavior:

Why I'm Unwilling to Adopt It:

Play in the Gray:

Sub-Behavior:

Why I'm Unwilling to Adopt It:

Play in the Gray:

Sub-Behavior:
Why I'm Unwilling to Adopt It:
Play in the Gray:

Pick a date to start practicing these sub-behaviors and write it here:

_____

Reflect for a moment on why you chose that date:

Are you satisfied you chose the right date? If not, then change the date you put down to one that makes more sense to you.

Viola! Done!

That wasn't so bad, was it?

It's actually a pretty easy process:

- Identify what behaviors will bring you the easiest success.
- Define what that behavior would be like when adopted successfully – this defines your sub-behaviors.
- Determine which of those sub-behaviors you are and are not willing to adopt right now.
- Play in the gray and modify the sub-behaviors until they are something you *are* willing to adopt.
- Set a date to take action.

Change doesn't have to be scary or hard, after all. This is your journey, which means *you* are in control.

Throughout your journey you are going to discover that some of the changes you thought would benefit you, actually don't. You'll also think of additional changes that you didn't capture initially. Both possibilities are awesome!

You are in control.

Reflect and adapt as necessary to ensure your success. Then, if you find yourself avoiding or resisting some of the changes you've determined are necessary, come back to this chapter and work through the willingness process to see why you are resisting, and what changes you can make to the behavior in order to adopt it willingly. Remember, you are now living in a gray world in which perfection is not an expectation—improvement is. Improvement means constant evaluation, change, soul-searching, and evolution. A decision you make today may not be the one you make tomorrow, and that's just the way the journey should be.

> This is your journey,
> which means you are in control.

CHAPTER 4

Self-Compassion and Accountability

Chapter 3 set you up to begin making important changes in your life and help you to overcome your life-long fight with emotional eating. You are now equipped to take action, but before you do, I want to talk about the importance of balancing accountability with self-compassion to create a successful and positive journey.

I want to tell you a little story.

Once upon a time, there was a bright, outgoing and precocious child named Sam. Sam was from China and moved to the United States at the tender age of eight. Sam was very excited to start school and make friends since it was pretty lonely living in a new place without any friends. Once Sam got to school there was an immediate road block to that goal; Sam didn't speak any English! So, Sam decided to work really hard and learn English quickly. Sam paid close attention during class and then studied and practiced English at home. When Sam started to practice speaking English with the other kids they laughed because the words were used all wrong. A little embarrassed but still determined, Sam decided to study harder. Trying again, Sam tried talking to the other boys and girls at school, only to be made fun of for using the wrong words at the wrong time. Feeling a bit deflated and lonely, Sam went home and practiced talking over and over again, making sure to get the words right. The next time Sam tried to talk to the kids at school, they scoffed at Sam's accent. This made Sam sad, frustrated and angry. There was just no winning! Did they realize how hard it was to learn English?! Did it have to be perfect for them to be friendly and talk back? Why work so hard to learn such a complicated language if no one was going to be nice or friendly?

At that point Sam gave up and decided to act sick in order to avoid going to school. It was just too frustrating and painful to continue to be rejected that way day after day. After a few days, Sam's parents figured out that Sam wasn't really sick and was just acting so they put Sam in a timeout for lying in order to skip school. This made Sam even angrier at the unfairness of it all. When forced back to school, Sam refused to participate in class and sat unresponsively until each day ended. The bright, outgoing, precocious child that moved to the US quickly turned into a quiet, apathetic, introverted child as a result of the constant rejection from the other students.

Breaks your heart, doesn't it?

Where were the encouragement, support, help, and acceptance that would have encouraged Sam rather than knock him down? Where was the compassion for working so hard, alone, on a difficult journey? What was the benefit of constantly berating Sam for not being perfect? With all of the ridicule, it was no wonder Sam gave up and quit the goal! Why work so hard if you are only going to be criticized?

Go look in a mirror. I mean it—get up, bring your book with you and look in the mirror. Don't worry, I'll wait.

You are looking at Sam.

Now, look harder... you are also looking at those mean other children.

Think about the words you say to yourself. How often do you call yourself stupid for making a simple mistake? How often do you call yourself weak or pathetic because you weren't perfect about sticking to a diet? How often do you call yourself ugly because you aren't a size _____?

So, let me repeat my earlier questions. Where are the encouragement, support, help and acceptance that would encourage you rather than knock you down? Where is the compassion for working so hard on a difficult journey? What is the benefit of constantly berating yourself for not being perfect? Why work so hard if you are only going to criticized yourself?

Who wants to continue a journey fraught with negativity, criticism, humiliation, and disgust? No one. That's absolutely no fun, and in fact it is demoralizing.

The simple truth is that for every negative thing you say about yourself or to yourself, you are setting yourself up to quit the journey. Is that what you want?

If not, are you willing to stop talking negatively to yourself and about yourself?

This is a good time to stop and journal because I don't want a flippant response to that last question. For some of you, stopping your emotional eating is going to be very, very tough to change. I want to support you, and teach you how to support yourself. The one person who is always there for you, is YOU. So, get out your notebook or fire up your computer, and start writing or typing. You might be surprised at what you learn about yourself.

While journaling, there are a few questions that I want you to answer:

1. Why do you feel compelled to speak negatively about/to yourself?
2. What comfort or protection do you gain from speaking negatively about/to yourself?
3. Are you conscious of how often you speak negatively about/to yourself?
4. Can you see the consequences of constantly berating yourself, despite successes?
5. Are you willing to change your self-dialogue no matter how imperfect your journey is? If not, why not?

Did any "a ha's" come out of this journaling exercise?

Sam's story has a few parallels to my own. When I was 10 years old, my parents and I moved from New Jersey to Florida. When we lived in New Jersey, life was awesome! I had my three older brothers still living with me, whom I idolized, my mom was the head of almost every organization in town (PTA, Girl Scouts, church organizations— you name it), I had a ton of hobbies from ballet to ice skating, gymnastics to girl scouts, and the neighborhood worked together to raise all the kids, so I was able to run free knowing I was safe and being monitored by someone nearby. In that type of environment I was happy, confident, and carefree with lots of friends.

All of that changed when we moved. My brothers were all old enough to go their own way, so none of them moved with us. We moved to a town that was made up primarily of retirees, so there were very few kids in my neighborhood to play with. My mom decided to take a break from leading so many organizations, limiting herself to just getting involved with the church, so she didn't meet as many other moms. There was obviously no opportunity to pursue ice skating, which was my favorite hobby, and the dance studios were not even close to the caliber of the ones in New Jersey. Each of these factors impacted my ability to meet and make friends with the kids in that town. When I finally started school, it never occurred to me that the kids wouldn't like me; as the sweetheart of my town in New Jersey I'd never experienced true rejection before. Well, I definitely experienced it then. It was pretty traumatizing and made for a lonely childhood fraught with uncertainty. Although I made friends, I would suddenly be rejected by them at some point with no warning and no explanation as to why. I was never sure when I was going to be rejected next. This brought on a number of insecurities I never had before. Feeling confident that I was a good person on the inside, I focused on my weight as the culprit for why I wasn't accepted.

You see, all of my life, I had watched and listened to my mom belittle and berate herself because she was overweight. She was and still is an amazing woman, but she acted as if she had no worth because she was overweight. For her, her only identity, her only value, was her size. So, if she wasn't worthy of love and acceptance, no matter what a wonderful woman she was, simply because she was overweight, then I figured that must be the answer for me as well, since I was also a good person who couldn't find love and acceptance among the kids at school.

That line of thinking brought on some pretty negative changes to my behaviors. Besides turning to anorexia, I also adopted the practice of publicly critiquing myself for every little thing. Being critiqued (aka rejected) by others was very painful for me, so I figured if I did it first they wouldn't feel the need to fire any shots at me. And, once again, this is what my mom did, and she was the person I loved and looked up to more than anyone else in the world. So, starting at the tender age of 11, I started verbally beating myself up on a regular basis until it was so habitual that I didn't even know I was doing it.

I now understand it was a form of protection from being rejected by others, but in truth, it simply encouraged me to reject myself. And that's exactly what ended up happening. I ended up in this constant state of self-rejection. No matter what I accomplished in life, it was never good enough; I constantly critiqued myself and tore myself down. Although that made for a very stressful, negative, self-defeating state of being, it was also comfortable and safe because I felt like I was protecting myself and pushing myself to always be better. However, this constant state of rejection caused me to fight my way through cyclical bouts of depression, exhaustion, anxiety, isolation, and binging.

You may be surprised to hear that I still have to work on this today. In fact, it wasn't until I met my boyfriend seven years ago that he made me aware of how often I beat myself up verbally. Even worse, it was so natural and so ingrained in me, that I didn't see anything wrong with it. How sad is that? I would call myself stupid or dumb or weak or fat at any provocation and I DIDN'T SEE ANYTHING WRONG WITH IT! Luckily, my man loved me more than I loved myself and wouldn't tolerate the negative self-talk. Anytime I would say something bad about myself, knowingly or not, he would stop me and simply say, "Try again" in that patient voice of his. After months of consistently being told "try again," I realized how often I berated myself and started to change my self-dialogue.

What comes out of our mouths becomes our truth, so it is very important to say and think what we want to believe. If you want to be self-confident, capable, intelligent, and attractive then you can't call yourself the opposite.

This is the first step towards showing self-compassion—changing your self-dialogue from negative to positive. Now, don't get me wrong. I don't want you saying things you don't believe; however,

I don't want you beating yourself up either. For example, when I've spent too many days indulging in sweet treats here or there and see a bloated version of myself in the mirror, I will no longer say, "God, look how fat I am! Ugh, that's disgusting!" Instead, I'll focus on aspects of my body that I like and say, "I have great hair and a great smile! I want to say that about the rest of me too. So, starting today I'm back on track and will love my body through food."

I'm not about to say "I'm beautiful" or "I'm looking fit and lean" when I don't believe it. That's simply lying. However, I'm not going to beat myself up about it either. That would simply encourage me to feel guilty, which in turn would encourage me to binge, and that isn't helpful at all. Self-compassion is recognizing and accepting that we aren't perfect and not letting that bring us down. Self-compassion is forgiving ourselves for being human and making mistakes. Self-compassion is treating ourselves the way we would treat a dear friend in the same situation we are in.

To start the process of demonstrating self-compassion, I want you to pay attention to what you say to yourself in your head as well as out loud for the next two days. There's no need to change it just yet. Simply pay attention, and get an idea of how often you berate yourself or speak negatively about yourself. Pay attention to how you handle compliments and successes. Pay attention to how you handle challenges and "failure." Start by simply paying attention.

Don't move forward with this chapter until you've completed this two-day exercise.

So, what did you learn in the last two days?

What situations caused you to speak negatively about yourself?

Were there any negative phrases you said to yourself or about yourself more often than others?

What are you willing to say instead of those phrases that are more positive, compassionate, and encouraging?

| |
| |
| |
| |
| |
| |
| |
| |
| |
| |
| |

Now, I want you to make a commitment—not to me, but to yourself—that you will begin the process of actively changing your self-dialogue from berating to self-compassionate. Let's make this a positive, inspiring journey rather than a grueling one, shall we?

With the art of self-compassion must also come the art of accountability. We need to maintain balance between the two in order to have both a happy and successful journey. Some of you may find that challenging because you don't know how to hold yourself accountable without tearing yourself down.

Let's start by defining accountability.

What is your definition of accountability?

How can you hold yourself accountable while still remaining self-compassionate?

I define accountability as holding myself responsible for both my successes and failures by acknowledging them when they occur and creating an action plan to either sustain or improve those results going forward. So, when I do things well, I acknowledge them and ensure I'm set up for continued success going forward. When I don't do things well, I acknowledge I need to make a change and then come up with a new game plan. What I DON'T do is beat myself up, tear myself down, or talk negatively to myself.

Here is a great example. Sundays are my days to get ready for a successful week of eating. I plan meals, do my grocery shopping and cook for the week so I am prepared and ready to go with very little work or thought needed during my work days. Recently, I've been spending most of my weekends out of town, so I don't have the ability to get myself ready for the week. That can easily lead me astray on my journey, which messes with my mind, body and spirit. No bueno!

Each Sunday night following an entire weekend out of town, I have to have a conversation with myself. Here is what that conversation *used* to sound like before I changed my self-dialogue.

"Ugh! You did it again! You can't keep going out of town each weekend and leaving yourself unprepared for the week. What are you going to do now? The stores are closed so you can't shop now, and you have clients starting at 5 a.m. tomorrow! Did you think of that before taking off? Of course not! You just took off, irresponsibly, and now look at where you're at! Why do you keep doing this to yourself? God, you're so stupid and stubborn! You just can't afford to take an entire weekend off when you have a business to run. You need to be more responsible! Now you're just going to cycle between starvation and binging because you don't have any food to eat. Nice job!"

Yikes! Pretty harsh, right? That conversation sounds exactly like what a mean kid would say to poor Sam. Luckily, I've changed my ways and have remodeled my conversations with myself. Here's what a typical Sunday night conversation with myself sounds like *now*:

"I'm glad that I spent the weekend enjoying my life! I work hard and am proud of the fact I am creating a better work/life balance in the midst of a stressful career! *(I start with this because I have a tendency to feel guilty for enjoying myself instead of working, so I need the reminder that I have permission to enjoy life.)* Now, I need to create a game plan for having a successful food week so that I don't stress out, feel fat, and feel like a failure on my lifetime journey. I need to keep perspective and live in the gray. My plan doesn't have to be perfect; it simply needs to set me up for success. Think healthy, balanced, and convenient. Think whole grain cereal with almond milk, Trader Joe's premade salads, and KIND bars with fruit. I've so got this!"

Big difference, right? You can see why I would feel compelled to binge after the original conversation and why I would feel empowered after the remodeled conversation. That's the point! We want to feel encouraged, supported, and empowered as a result of our self-dialogue, not torn down, beat up and berated. The balance of accountability and self-compassion is not allowing yourself to make excuses for failure, but instead acknowledging the situation without judgment or guilt, and creating a logical go-forward strategy you can implement immediately.

Like Sam, you deserve encouragement, support, help, and acceptance as you work on the most important change of your life. If you commit to treating yourself with self-compassion while holding yourself accountable for implementing the changes we discuss in this book, you will have a much higher chance of long-term success on this journey. It is much easier to remain motivated in a positive, supportive environment than a negative, self-defeating one.

CHAPTER 5

Eating for Nutrition, not Weight Loss

Since each of you will be tackling your behaviors in a different order, I'm going to spend the rest of the book going through the behaviors in the order I introduced them in Chapter 1. You can either skip to the chapters that cover the behaviors you plan to tackle first and then come back to the others, or follow the book, as written. As I mentioned in the last chapter, this is your journey, so you are in control.

Since Chapters 1-3 tackled the first behavior, getting the right mindset and setting realistic expectations for the journey, this chapter will focus on the second and third behaviors: Eating for health, nutrition and enjoyment, not weight loss.

Let's be realistic. If health and nutrition were our only concerns, we would have changed our eating habits a long time ago. But enjoyment is pretty important and provides the immediate gratification we all crave, so that's got to stay in the picture, as well, if we want long-term success. So, how do we balance the two?

First, we need to define what is healthy and nutritious, then we can figure out how to make it delicious. I'm going to let my inner geek come out and hope I don't scare you away. I'll try to keep the science as simple as possible, because in order to understand how to make healthier food choices, you need to understand what "healthy" means.

You may have heard the term "macros," but many of you may not know what that really means. Macros is an abbreviation for macronutrients. Carbohydrates (aka carbs), fats and proteins are macronutrients. Macros are the three main nutrients in our diet we must have in LARGE amounts to survive. And although science is always changing, this is one fact that has not yet changed. This means that neither carbs nor fats are bad, despite what you've heard in the media. They each have a purpose in our diet. The only question you need to answer is how much of each does YOUR body need to feel, look and act its best?

And only YOU can answer that. Do you feel energized or lethargic after a meal? Do you feel lean or bloated after a meal? Do you get heartburn or stomach troubles after a meal? Do you have the energy you need to get your work and hobbies done each day, or do you run out of energy midday? These are all questions you should ask yourself to figure out what combination of macros works best for you.

Although the right balance of macros is the first vital element of health and nutrition, the second is your micronutrients. Micronutrients are the nutrients we need in small amounts to survive. Micronutrients are the vitamins and minerals you get from your food. Both macronutrients and micronutrients are VITAL not only for our survival, but our quality

> Macronutrients = Carbs, Proteins and Fats
>
> Micronutrients = Vitamins and Minerals
>
> Both are vital to our survival and quality of life

of life, as well. The more you nourish your body with the "good" stuff, the more efficiently your body will run, the less disease and injury you'll have to fight, and the more energy you'll have.

So, what does that look like? Although many people don't trust the government, their MyPlate recommendations (from the USDA, see https://www.choosemyplate.gov/MyPlate) are actually a pretty good place to start! Here's the simple version: ladies, choose a salad plate; gentlemen, choose a dinner plate. Then, fill half your plate with fruits and vegetables (more vegetables than fruit), a quarter of your plate with whole grains, and the other quarter of your plate with lean protein. They also recommend a glass of milk on the side, which you can take or leave based on your opinions about dairy and any allergies you may have. Overall, the recommendations promote reasonable portion sizes and nutritional balance, which are keys to both health and weight loss.

Obviously, as a health coach, I am asked about weight loss a lot. So, I want to give a little more insight into the MyPlate recommendations with my own little spin on it. Here is what I recommend:

1. Eat food in the proper portion sizes.
   a. Your body can only digest and absorb so much at one time. Anything beyond that will be stored as fat.
   b. If you don't want to change WHAT you eat, change HOW MUCH you eat. Cut everything you currently eat in half and save the other half for another meal 3-4 hours later. So, if you currently eat a Big Mac with a large order of french fries and a large Coke™, I recommend that you cut that Big Mac in half, choose a small order of fries and a small Coke™ and save the other half of the burger until later. That alone will help you lose weight.
2. Eat whole foods.
   a. In general, the more processed a food is, the less micronutrients or vitamins and minerals it has.
   b. I believe your body has an easier time digesting, absorbing and utilizing foods in their natural state because it recognizes what the food is and what to do with it. Therefore, it doesn't have much left over to store as fat. Processed foods, on the other hand, are seen as foreign substances by the body, and if the

body doesn't know what to do with the stuff, it simply stores it as fat. Fat isn't very biased; it'll take anything you give it, so if the body isn't sure what to do with a certain food, it sends it over to the fat who happily accepts it and places it on your belly and hips.

3. Determine the amount of carbs you need based on your activity level.

    a. What are examples of healthy carbs? Whole grains, whole grain breads, whole grain pastas, fruits, vegetables, and legumes. Basically, anything that is not a fat or protein is a carbohydrate. If you have a very active job or exercise intensely for over an hour each day, the amount of carbs you eat, and specifically grain-based carbs, should be higher because your body needs energy for all of that activity.

    b. If you have a sedentary job but you exercise pretty intensely each day, then you should eat a moderate amount of grain-based carbs.

    c. If you are pretty sedentary overall and do minimal exercise, you should eat a low amount of grain-based carbs, because your body doesn't need as much energy.

4. Eat three-five times per day.

    a. Some people hate snacking or don't have time for it. If that is the case, ensure you at least eat a good breakfast, lunch and dinner.

    b. If you have more than a four-hour gap between meals, I recommend having a healthy snack in between the two to keep your metabolism fired up, and to keep you from getting overly hungry and binging when you finally have time to eat your next meal.

That's it—to start. Of course, there are a number of other things you can do for health, nutrition and weight loss, but these four guidelines are a great start and provide enough guidance to really make a difference in both your health and your physique. Remember, we want to find a healthy way to eat that we can sustain for the long haul, which means anything too restrictive or complicated won't work. These four guidelines are simple, easy to remember and easy to do. And since this topic can fill an entire book (book number 2, maybe?) I'm going to stick with the basics so it won't distract us from our real objective of overcoming emotional eating.

But that only covers eating for health and nutrition. What about enjoying your food? I believe enjoying your food is as important to your success as following the four guidelines. If the food you eat is consistently boring or tasteless, you are going to go back to your old eating habits quickly. So, we

> 4 Nutritional/Weight Loss Recommendations:
>
> 1. Eat proper portion sizes
> 2. Eat whole foods
> 3. Choose number of carbs based on activity level
> 4. Eat 3-5x per day

need to figure out how to make the delicious nutritious, and vice versa.

There are two primary ways to make food nutritious and two primary ways to make food delicious:

Nutritious	Delicious
1. Choose whole foods	1. Make things flavorful
2. Include a variety of colors	2. Create a pleasing texture

Simple enough, right?

Let's take pizza as an example. Most of the fat and calories of a pizza come from the crust, cheese and processed meat toppings. So, can you still eat pizza? YES! Just differently. I recommend ordering thin crust (crispy texture), light cheese (gooey texture), red (tomato) sauce (flavor), as many vegetable toppings as you want (color and whole foods) and then maybe some sliced ham (flavor) or chicken breast (whole food) if you want some meat on there. Your pizza will be both nutritious and delicious! Then, watch your portion sizes (maybe order a smaller sized pizza) when it arrives at your table and you can feel really good about eating pizza while remaining healthy and losing weight!

Is it *as* delicious or decadent as your favorite pizza? No, it's not, but your favorite pizza has made you the size you are today and you purchased this book because you want to be a different size in the future. So, you've got to make some changes to what you are doing today in order to achieve your goals tomorrow.

Here's another example that takes a bit more work, but it satisfies my craving for sausage, which I LOVE! It's my favorite food, but definitely not a food that is considered nutritious or helpful in losing weight. Although chicken and turkey sausages are lower in fat, they can have nasty fillers in them and get really dried out when you cook them. What's a girl to do!?!? Make her own, that's what! I make my own breakfast sausage patties and they are delicious! Here are my ingredients:

Theresa's Sausages

- 1lb ground chicken breast
- 1 mashed avocado
- ½ steamed sweet potato, mashed
- Sausage seasoning mix (make your own – easy to find a recipe online)
- ½ box/bag frozen, thawed and drained chopped spinach

The chicken breast is a lean protein source that is minimally processed in comparison to actual sausage. The spinach provides color, vitamins, minerals, and believe it or not, texture. The spinach also helps keep the sausage patties moist rather than dried out and doesn't mess with the flavor. The sweet potato acts as a healthy binder for the sausage and helps add the sweetness I love in breakfast sausage. The avocado provides that fatty texture we all know and love in sausage, and yet it is healthy. And, of course, the sausage seasoning mix ensures my sausage is bursting with flavor. I mix this all together, form ¼-pound patties and cook them in a skillet using a non-stick spray. Viola! Whole foods, a variety of colors, flavors, and a real sausage-like texture and it doesn't take that long to make. I couldn't be happier to wake up to that in the morning!

Making the nutritious delicious and the delicious nutritious takes some work, but if it can improve your health and help you lose weight, isn't it worth it? Actually, once again, only you can decide that. I know that for me, it definitely is!

So, as you move forward creating deliciously nutritious meals, don't hesitate to steal ideas! There are so many great food blogs on the internet, as well as a plethora of recipes on Pinterest. Below are some of my favorite food blogs to grab healthy ideas from, and this is a small list in comparison to all of the favorites I have saved. Please note that not all the recipes on these websites are weight loss friendly, so continue to choose wisely despite my recommendations.

Iowa Girl Eats
Ambitious Kitchen
Minimalist Baker
Budget Bytes
Damn Delicious
All Recipes
Menu Musings
Half Baked Harvest

CHAPTER 6

Eating Mindfully

Eating deliciously nutritious meals helps improve our health and ability to lose weight, but doesn't really help us tackle our root problem. So, let's discuss a behavior that impacts both weight loss *and* emotional eating: Mindless eating. You know, those times when the repetitive motion of hand-to-mouth is so comforting, and you don't even realize you are doing it? Yup, that's the quintessential description of mindless eating.

For me it sneaks up on long car rides, in front of the TV, hanging out with my girlfriends, or when I'm bored out of my mind.

Mindless eating is a key contributor to being overweight and is a bad habit for many emotional eaters. For some of us, it is an oral fixation in which we unconsciously find comfort with the repetitive action of hand-to-mouth. For others, it is simply a habit that we fall back on when we are bored or feeling emotional. The problem is that there is no thought or consideration while we are mindlessly eating, hence the name. There are times we have no idea we are even eating! At other times we consciously make the decision to eat, but then get lost in the action and forget to stop. Either way, it is detrimental to our emotional, spiritual, and physical health, so we need to get control of it.

As I'm sure you've noticed by now, I'm a "take action" kinda gal. So, instead of just talking about it, we are going to work towards solving it—right now.

Let's start by identifying the situations in which you eat mindlessly. I have no doubts you'll add to this list as you start paying attention to your eating habits, but this is a good place to start.

Mindless Eating Situations:

| |
| |
| |
| |
| |
| |
| |
| |
| |

As I mentioned earlier, you'll probably add to this list as you pay more attention to your eating habits. A really good way to become more aware of your habits is to keep a food log for a week.

Okay, I may have just lost some of you on that one...but notice I said only for **a week**.

I am a huge believer in food logging and have been keeping a daily food log for over 15 years. It is one of the tools I use to keep me honest and mindful, and as a result I have kept off the 45 pounds I lost 15 years ago. Because I love making lists, food logging is natural and easy for me. However, I know that isn't the case for many of you, and THAT'S OKAY!!!! I don't believe you should do what I do simply because it works for me. I think you need to figure out what works for you.

Having said that, I still recommend keeping a food log for one week in order to become more aware of your eating habits. Based on my experience with my clients, the majority honestly believe they know what they eat on a day-to-day basis, and then are shocked silly when they actually start logging everything they eat. It is amazing how many "bites" or "tastes" you can take in a day that you happily "forget" when reviewing your day. Emotional eaters easily discount or forget bites and tastes, as if those calories don't count. Unfortunately, they do count, and can seriously impact both your weight and your mindless eating habit.

So, for those of you who hate the idea of food logging, try it for only one week so you can see what's what. Needless to say, if you change your habits for that week so you don't have to write down anything "bad" the effort will be for naught, so just keep doing what you've been doing. No one is going to see your log. No one is going to judge you. And really, the only person you'll hurt is yourself and you've done enough of that already. The whole purpose of this book is to stop hurting yourself and start loving yourself. So, be honest and give yourself the opportunity to take the right action steps to heal your life.

Before you jump into action, let's review a variety of ways you can successfully log your food. There are a variety of apps you can use, such as My Fitness Pal, Fat Secret, or Spark People, just to name a few. The benefit of using apps like these is being able to see your calorie and macro breakdown. The drawback is the amount of time it takes to find or add your food in their extensive databases. Another method is simply carrying a small notebook with you and writing down when and what you eat throughout the day. The benefit of using a notebook is that it is easy and quick; the drawback is that you have to carry something around with you all day long. I, personally, use a Notes app on my phone. It is easy like a notebook, but I don't have to carry anything additional around with me all day.

These are only a few examples of how to log your food, but no matter the method, the information that will help you the most is:

- What you ate
- How much you ate
- When you ate
- How it was cooked (ex: fried, boiled, baked, etc)

If you capture this information for a week, you will have much greater insight into your eating habits on weekdays and weekend days.

This is a good time to put this book down, take a week to log your food and figure out your eating trends, and then continue reading this chapter. See you in a week! ☺

Welcome back! Have you gained any insights into your eating habits?

Hopefully, the food logging assignment helped you identify the times in your life when you eat mindlessly the most often. Now, you can pay more attention to what you are doing. It is so much harder to continue bad habits when we become aware of them, which is why awareness is always the first step. ☺

Obviously, if we want to stop eating mindLESSLY, we need to do the opposite and start eating mindFULLY.

Eating mindfully simply means making a conscious decision about whether you should or should not eat or drink something before you eat or drink it. That's it!

Eating mindfully does not mean you will no longer eat in the situations you listed above. It simply means you are going to make a conscious decision to eat **something delicious and nutritious when you are hungry** in the situations you listed above. As you know, there's no need for an emotional eater to be hungry when we eat. All we need is the desire to eat and we can eat nonstop for hours. That's the habit we are going to break.

So, for example, I hate driving. To me, driving is boring and a waste of time. I have things to do at point A and things to do at point B and driving is simply a necessary evil to get me to my destination. I also have very little patience for other drivers, so driving is a very frustrating affair for me. Needless to say, this is a prime situation for me to eat mindlessly. Eating while driving is both comforting and distracting. It also keeps me awake when I have to drive long distances. I don't sit well, and sitting for long periods of time typically puts me to sleep—not a good combination when driving. So, because I now live in this beautiful gray world filled with lots of options, I have come up with a list of healthy snacks I'm willing to have with me when I drive. It's important to note that just because I have them with me doesn't mean I'm automatically going to eat them—that's still eating mindlessly, just with healthier foods. No,

I am still going to make a conscious decision of whether or not to snack while I drive.

"So, Theresa, what does it mean to make a conscious decision whether to eat or not?" I am so glad you asked!

I have come up with what I call the S.A.C.K. method for overcoming mindless eating. I want to sack my bad habits, so it seemed appropriate! ☺

When I get the urge to eat, I:

> **S**top! – Stop for a full 30 seconds before taking the first bite. This forces me to think. Thirty seconds is a long time when you really just want to start eating, but I put myself on the clock, and I recommend you do the same. Your phone has a timer on it. Have it automatically set to 30 seconds and hit "Start" when you have a craving.

During those 30 seconds:

> **A**nalyze why you want to eat and whether you will feel good about it when you are finished eating. I do this by stating my goal in my head. For example, "I want to lose five pounds by the end of this month." Then, I ask myself, "Will this help or hinder my ability to hit my goal?" Based on my answer, I know what to do. If, during this analysis, I realize I haven't eaten in three hours and I am actually hungry, then yes, eating will help me hit my weight loss goal. And by having healthier snacks on hand, I can feel good about what I eat.

> How to Overcome Mindless Eating:
> **The S.A.C.K. Method**
>
> S – Stop
> A – Analyze
> C – Commit
> K – Kudos

Once you've analyzed the situation, then:

> **C**ommit to the decision without feeling guilty. For example, let's say you are craving chocolate and after stopping for 30 seconds and analyzing your craving, you decide that you can afford a piece of chocolate. Eat it, enjoy it, and don't feel guilty about it! Commit to your decision because it was a mindful one. There is no reason for guilt at that point. If you start feeling guilty, you give that food power over you which may set off a binge. Don't allow that!

So instead of guilt, I want you to give yourself:

> **K**udos – We are so used to beating ourselves up when it comes to food and our eating habits. We need to change that. Instead, we need to make food and eating a positive experience. If you have worked your way through the SAC method, you deserve some kudos for breaking an unhealthy habit, adopting a healthy habit, and sticking with it. Although these methods are simple, they aren't easy, and we need to acknowledge the efforts we are making. For some of you, this will be the toughest step of the S.A.C.K. method—but that doesn't give you permission to skip it! If you want to love yourself, then you need to treat yourself with love. You deserve to love and respect yourself. Go for it!

That's it!

Stop
Analyze
Commit
Kudos

Although this is a simple way to become more mindful, it's only beneficial if you actually use it. To make this a habit, go through the SACK method each time you eat or drink ANYTHING during the next two weeks and see how it works for you. If you can make the SACK method a habit, eating mindlessly will become a thing of the past, and wouldn't that just be awesome?!?! One less bad habit keeping you away from being a healthy, happy individual—yay!

CHAPTER 7

Praise Phrase

As I mentioned in the last chapter, giving yourself kudos is an important and positive step on your journey towards overcoming emotional eating. Now is a good time to discuss the importance of recognizing and acknowledging our successes at all times, and not just when we are using the S.A.C.K. method. To build our self-confidence we have to do more than stop pointing out all of our faults and failings. We need to praise ourselves for the things we have done well.

Stop and think about that for a second. I want you to actively praise yourself throughout the day; not just when you make a good food choice, but *every single time* you do something well.

What is your immediate reaction to that idea?

| |
| |
| |
| |
| |

As children, many of us were taught to be modest and not to brag; for many of us who grew up in a religious household, we were taught that pride is a sin! We were taught to downplay our successes and act as if they weren't important; modesty was approved of and pride frowned upon. So, for many of us, minimizing our achievements is a lifelong habit.

Although it may be tough, it's time to break that habit!

Remember Sam? Just think how well Sam would have done with a bit of praise and acknowledgment. If someone had only said, "Good job, Sam! Your English is getting better every day! Keep up the good work!" Sam would have persevered with learning English and felt proud of the continued improvements despite making little grammatical mistakes.

That's what you need to do for yourself. Praise yourself and acknowledge what you do well despite little mistakes here and there. You aren't meant to be perfect on this journey, just better. So, praise yourself every time you are better! This practice isn't limited to your actions regarding your health. Praising yourself is something you should practice in all areas of your life, from parenting to your job to your weight loss journey.

Although I'm sure there are multiple ways to go about acknowledging your successes, I'm going to focus on what works well for me, and that's using a "praise phrase."

As a child (and even now as an adult ☺), my mom would always praise me with the words, "Good girl!" I knew that my mom was proud of me and happy with whatever I said or did when she told me "good girl!" As a result, when I was thinking of what I could say to myself to acknowledge my successes, I immediately thought of, "good girl!" Those two words bring a warm sensation to my chest because with them comes the feelings of safety, approval, love, and pride that I felt from my mom when she said them. Those two words seemed like the perfect praise phrase to use when I wanted to acknowledge my success in any area of my life. This is the phrase I use when I give myself kudos during the S.A.C.K. method.

What will your praise phrase be?

I am a big believer in keeping things simple and authentic, so I recommend that you use something quick and easy that sparks feelings of self-satisfaction and pride when you say it to yourself.

Write your praise phrase here:

_____

_____

Now, here's where the fun or the hard part comes in, depending on your perspective. You have to say it to yourself! Every single time you do something well, use your praise phrase.

The other day I really, really, really wanted a pumpkin chocolate chip bar. (I made them the previous week and they were just screaming my name!) Despite the fact that the bars were made with healthy ingredients, I just didn't need it and I wasn't actually hungry. I just wanted something sweet. So, I fought off the craving and distracted myself with some other activity. Twenty minutes later, when I realized I had successfully avoided giving into a craving, I gave myself a silent yet very exuberant "good girl!" in my head.

That one is a pretty obvious example. Here's a less obvious one.

I've been trying to get in the habit of taking fish oil capsules each day because of all the health benefits I can gain from taking them. Unfortunately, I hate taking capsules and these are HUGE, and they make me nauseous. I'm not willing to swallow fish oil as a liquid, so there's little I can do about the size of the capsules. To avoid the nausea, I have started taking them at night before bed so that I sleep through the nausea. (Brilliant, I know...ha ha. ☺)

The problem is, this is a new practice for me, so I often forget to take the damn things. Even with the bottle sitting on my night stand, I'll forget and just conk out for the night. So, each night that I *do* remember to take them I give myself a "good girl." New habits are hard to adopt, so I need to acknowledge every success and keep myself motivated to continue to take the fish oil capsules. I know that eventually I won't even have to think about it, but I'm not there yet. So, I will continue to encourage myself with my praise phrase every time I remember to take the capsules.

Now, it's your turn. I want you to think about the various instances throughout the day when you can and should use your praise phrase to acknowledge your successes, big and small. What can you praise yourself for?

Here are some ideas, if you didn't already think of them.

- Every time you take a drink of water to stay hydrated
- Every time you go to bed early enough to get a full night's sleep
- Every time you wake up early to get yourself mentally, spiritually and emotionally ready for the day
- Every time you eat something nutritious
- Every time you stick to your meal plan
- Every time you take the time to plan a meal
- Every time you order something healthier than you normally would at a restaurant
- Every time you only eat half of your order at a restaurant
- Every time you eat your healthy snack during the day
- Every time you journal
- Every time you do something to enhance your health
- Every time you do something nice for someone else
- Every time you do something nice for yourself
- Every time you are successful at work
- Every time you incorporate movement into your day

- Every time you help someone else succeed at their goal
- Every time you use the SACK method to overcome a craving or a binge
- Every time you actively change your self-dialogue from critiquing to positive
- Every time you are in tune with your hunger and consciously decide to eat or not to eat
- Every time you are civil/nice to the person at work who drives you crazy
- Every time you are patient with a child, customer, parent, sibling, etc. when you really just want to yell at them

See? There are plenty of opportunities to praise ourselves throughout each day.

Perhaps you may think that some of the options on the list are too mundane to be worthy of praise. If that's so, then why do we tear ourselves down over the same mundane things? How often have you torn yourself down because you didn't drink enough water that day? How often have you torn yourself down because you feel exhausted all the time and just don't seem to have the energy to do anything? How often do you tear yourself down for eating a snack that's not on your meal plan? If you can critique yourself for the mundane, you can also praise yourself for it.

Self-confidence comes from feeling pride in who we are and what we are able to accomplish despite our fears and challenges. The key words are "feeling pride." You can't feel pride in yourself if you are unwilling to acknowledge when you've been successful, so if you really want to be a self-confident person who is comfortable in your own skin, it's time to start looking for opportunities to feel proud of yourself—both big and small. This will make the journey you are on more fun, motivational, inspiring and positive. It will also help you to progress further and faster, so don't negate the importance of positivity.

Over the next week, I want you to focus on two things: eating mindfully and creating opportunities to use your praise phrase. I want you to use the S.A.C.K. method before putting ANYTHING in your mouth to help you successfully adopt this new habit, and to ensure that whatever you choose to eat is a good decision.

And, of course, if you work through all of the steps of the S.A.C.K. method throughout the day, you'll also be saying your praise phrase consistently throughout the day, as well. However, I want you to create OTHER opportunities to use your praise phrase outside of the S.A.C.K. method. I want you to say it multiple times for non-diet related reasons, throughout the day and see how you feel after a week of saying it to yourself.

If you recognize that you aren't saying your praise phrase very often, figure out what the barrier is that's stopping you from saying it.

- Are you not doing anything worth being proud of? That's doubtful.
- Are you resistant to the idea of praising yourself? Why?
- Are you unwilling to acknowledge the small successes and are waiting for a big success to use your praise phrase?
- What is the worst that could happen if you praised yourself often throughout the day?

Being willing to acknowledge your successes is a crucial step so you can experience a positive journey that creates feelings of self-worth and confidence. Feelings of success, self-worth and positivity will help you to stay on course and persevere through your journey of overcoming emotional eating, even in the face of challenges and setbacks.

CHAPTER 8

Negative Emotions and Food

The last two chapters have focused heavily on the importance of positive self-talk, whether it is as passive as simply not tearing yourself down or as active as praising yourself for each of your successes, big or small. Both are equally important to your journey. But in order to really use these new practices, we have to get a better grip on what it means to live in the world of gray. We talked about it briefly in Chapter 3, but now seems like a good time to delve a bit deeper into this new, gray world.

Life is not black and white. Food is not "good" or "bad." Actions are not "right" or "wrong." There are a lot of gray areas between each of those extremes.

> Food is not "good" or "bad." The moment we think of food as "bad" we give it a power it doesn't deserve.

When we live our lives from the perspective of extremes, we set ourselves up to constantly feel disappointed by our actions, which triggers our self-disgust, which triggers an eating binge, which triggers more guilt, which triggers more self-disgust, which triggers another binge, which triggers more guilt. You get the picture.

An important key to remaining positive during this journey is keeping our perspective so that we don't make judgments about or invest our emotions in things that don't deserve them.

For example, a brownie is not bad. The moment we think of a brownie as "bad," we give it power that it doesn't deserve to have. That brownie now has the power to make us feel guilt, to make us feel self-disgust, to make us feel fat, etc., when in truth a brownie is simply 250-300 calories of flour, eggs, sugar and other ingredients that create a high energy snack. When you use the S.A.C.K. method in a gray world, you can enjoy the brownie and then create a plan for adding a bit more movement to your day (to burn those calories), or you can choose to eat fewer high energy calories later in the day to compensate for the brownie. It's not a big deal.

I repeat—IT'S NOT A BIG DEAL!

If we were in our old black and white world and we thought of that same brownie as "bad," we would feel guilty after eating it, and beat ourselves up mentally, which could easily trigger an eating binge, and that could cause us to eat the entire platter of brownies instead of just one.

Okay. THAT *IS* A BIG DEAL!

Just to be clear:

Eating one brownie = NOT A BIG DEAL.
Eating an entire platter of brownies = A BIG DEAL.

Very simple math.

It is very important that we truly embrace a world of gray, in which we take "good" and "bad" and "right" and "wrong" out of our vocabularies.

This concept often creates serious concerns and even fears in my clients. The most common concerns are:

"What is to stop me from eating cakes, cookies and chips if I no longer consider them to be bad?"

"Seeing certain foods as good and bad gives me boundaries. How can I expect to lose weight if I don't have any boundaries?"

"Shouldn't I feel bad when I eat something that works against my weight loss goal? I can't imagine *not* feeling bad when I eat something I'm not supposed to."

These questions lead to some really good points.

Binging "What is to stop me from eating cakes, cookies and chips if I no longer consider them to be bad?"

This first concern is typically based on the fear of binging. You don't trust your ability to stop at just one serving of whatever it is you deem "bad." You are terrified that if you allow yourself to eat a brownie you won't be able to stop eating until all the brownies are gone.

In this case, the brownie is what I call a trigger, a food that causes addiction-related chemicals to be released in your brain that limits your ability to control yourself. A trigger is similar to the way liquor or beer affects an alcoholic, or the way cocaine affects a drug addict. For some people this is a very valid fear—in which case you *do* need to look at that brownie differently. For you, a brownie is no longer a sweet treat but a drug. You may be addicted to sugar, or to carbohydrates in general.

If this fear resonates with you, then I want you to skip to the page 137 in Chapter 11 and work through the activities explained there. Chapter 11 is all about triggers and addictions. You can go back to the beginning of Chapter 11 after you work through the activities on page 137, but I think you should start there for the greatest impact and help on your journey.

Control "Seeing certain foods as good and bad gives me boundaries. How can I expect to lose weight if I don't have any boundaries?"

A concern about the need for boundaries is based on a fear of losing control. If this concern resonates with you, I suspect that you work best with structure in many facets of your life. You like having expectations and boundaries because they keep you on task. I am in this category, too. I thrive in structured situations and tend to fall apart in the absence of structure. The good news is that you can have structure and still live in a gray world! There are multiple ways to do it, and you can make different choices at different times and in different circumstances.

There are three primary techniques I fall back on:

- I only eat half of the treat and save the other half for another day.
- I save the treat until right after my workout, when I know my body will utilize all of those high energy calories.
- I enjoy my treat and then compensate by proportionately reducing the amount of carbohydrates and fat that I plan to eat during the rest of the day, or by adding in a workout.

I don't necessarily use all of these techniques at once, but I do determine which one(s) make the most sense for me at that moment. The key is that I will employ at least one of these techniques every time. That sets me up for success, because I have already thought about these techniques before I need to use them, and I can pick and choose which one I want to employ at the time rather than being so rigid.

Once again, these aren't the only techniques; these are simply *my* techniques. Be careful that any technique you choose to use does not set you up to fail. For example, if you decide that one of your techniques is to only have treats on special occasions, then you set yourself up to feel guilty if you have a treat when there is no "special occasion." A better technique is to limit yourself to three treats per week, or commit to exercising for a minimum of 30 minutes each time you eat a treat, or goals similar to that. That gives you boundaries and flexibility.

Since having your techniques ready before you need them is helpful for your success, take a few minutes and define what techniques you will use to create structure and boundaries around eating treats.

Your techniques for creating flexible structure with "treats"

Now that you have chosen what techniques you will use, you can enjoy treats—in moderation—without feeling guilty about it! Yay!

Guilt "Shouldn't I feel bad when I eat something that works against my weight loss goal? I can't imagine *not* feeling bad when I eat something I'm not supposed to."

Speaking of guilt, if this concern resonates most with you, then guilt is a key driver in your life. It is likely that you are easily manipulated as well as motivated by guilt. If you look at the definition of guilt in the Merriam-Webster dictionary it is defined as, "responsibility for a crime or for doing something bad or wrong," or "a bad feeling caused by knowing or thinking that you have done something bad or wrong." Guilt is a very strong emotion, and has a time and place, but I disagree that that time and place is with eating.

If you intentionally hurt someone or something, then it's appropriate to feel guilty. If you eat something responsibly that brings you pleasure, guilt is misplaced. You aren't doing anything bad or wrong; you aren't committing any crime; you aren't intentionally hurting yourself or someone else. What you are doing is experiencing pleasure, responsibly. Don't you deserve to feel pleasure and enjoy yourself?

I don't want you to gloss over that question but to take it seriously. Don't you deserve to feel pleasure and enjoy yourself?

Most people who suffer from frequent feelings of guilt also suffer from some form of self-loathing over some real or imagined transgression that they need to forgive themselves for. If you often feel guilty for even small, inconsequential things, it is time for you to do some soul searching and figure out what the root cause of that is—and then forgive yourself for it. Until you can forgive yourself, you won't be willing or able to stop feeling guilty, no matter what techniques I teach you.

Take some time and figure out the root cause of why you frequently feel guilty, and how you can forgive yourself for it, so you can finally release the guilt and move on with a healthy, self-loving life.

This makes me feel guilty:

This is how I can forgive myself:

Self-forgiveness is not always easy, so you may not be able to resolve this today. But, don't give up on it; continue to journal and soul search until you can work yourself into a place of forgiveness. Perpetual guilt is very heavy to bear; by forgiving yourself and letting go of all of that guilt you will allow all of the pressure, judgment, and self-loathing to be released from your shoulders.

Just to make sure the proper expectation is set, the last activity doesn't free you from ever feeling guilt. It simply allows you to feel guilt when it is appropriate, rather than all of the time.

For example, if you eat an entire plate of brownies, then you have intentionally hurt yourself. I want you to regret hurting yourself in that way. I don't want you to feel guilty because you are judging yourself as weak; I want you to feel guilty for HURTING yourself! There is a big difference between those two reasons for feeling guilt. Does that make sense to you? Eating a properly portioned treat is not what caused you to gain so much weight. Eating too many treats, or too much of a treat at a time is what caused you to gain so much weight. In this case, the activity on page 103 will help you to create the structure you need to continue to enjoy yourself without guilt while continuing to work successfully towards your weight loss goal.

That is the beauty of living in a gray world; you get to continue to enjoy the occasional treat without giving it the power to make you feel bad about it.

CHAPTER 9

Feeling Emotions

Okay, take a deep breath. This is going to be our deepest, probably most challenging chapter of the book. This is the chapter where we learn to feel, experience, and accept our emotions. For an emotional eater, that's damn scary. The whole reason we are emotional eaters is because we avoid feeling emotions that we think are too much for us to handle. As scary as it is, we need to overcome that fear in order to truly break our cycle of emotional eating.

I want to remind you that I'm not a therapist, nor am I trained in emotional counseling. I am an emotional eater who struggles with many of the same challenges you do. I am an emotional eater who has spent a lot of time soul-searching and figuring out what works best for me. In this chapter, I'm going to share tips and techniques that help me to overcome my fear of feeling, and techniques that help me learn to accept, experience, and release my emotions so that I no longer have to rely on food for comfort and distraction.

Let's start by talking about emotions and a very important lesson that I learned from Brené Brown. Brené Brown is a researcher, famous speaker, and bestselling author on the topics of courage, vulnerability,

> You can't limit one emotion without limiting them all.

empathy, and shame. She is the author of some of my favorite self-help books, including *Daring Greatly* and *The Gift of Imperfection*.

Through both her talks and her books, she taught me that I can't limit one emotion without limiting them all. So, if you refuse to experience the ultimate hurt and sadness, then you will never truly be able to feel the ultimate joy and happiness. Love and connection require vulnerability; vulnerability can often lead to feeling hurt. Many of us, who are afraid of such emotions, may struggle to feel the love and connection we so crave. To go through life never feeling the love and connection we deserve is tragic and completely unnecessary. That's simply an unconscious choice we make out of fear—the fear of being hurt or rejected. It's time to let go of that fear and begin really feeling so that we can begin really living!

Part of my fear of emotions is a fear of losing control. I like to feel in control, and I don't feel in control when I'm overrun by emotions. Let's take anger, for example. I feel both empowered and terrified by my anger. Anger is a powerful emotion because I feel strong, justified, and ready to fight for my rights. I have no fear of standing up for myself when I'm angry and I LOVE that about anger! However, it can also be a very destructive emotion that can cause hurt feelings, possibly physical harm, and severed relationships. It is an emotion that can cause a lot of feelings of guilt. That's the part I fear—losing control and doing or saying something I will regret. So, before I learned to deal with my anger, I would squelch it and eat instead.

Hurt is a completely different emotional experience for me. Hurt makes me feel vulnerable; it makes me want to run and hide. Instead of empowering me, it makes me feel weak, unloved, unwanted, and insecure. Who wants to feel that?! So, it makes sense that I'd want to avoid feeling that emotion and turn to the pleasant and distracting act of eating instead.

Although it makes sense, it clearly isn't the best choice for our mental, spiritual and physical health, so it's time to change that pattern and deal with ALL of our emotions, both "good" and "bad."

Since this is going to take some work, I'm going to break this chapter up into sections so we can tackle this one step at a time. Although this process isn't easy, I like to keep things as simple as possible.

Figure Out Why Emotions Scare You

Let's start by determining what it is about emotions that scares you. If scare isn't the right word, replace it with a more appropriate word, but don't let the wrong word stop you from getting the most out of this activity.

Here were some of the things that I wrote down when I completed this activity:

- I'm afraid to lose control.
- I'm afraid to feel/be vulnerable.
- I don't like conflict, so if I allow myself to feel hurt, disappointment, or anger I'll actually have to deal with it and the person that caused it.
- I'm afraid of what I'll learn about myself if I look too deep inside.
- I'm afraid of feeling devastated if I admit that someone I love or respect actually hurt me.
- I'm afraid I'll never stop crying if I start.
- I'm afraid that I won't feel anything, and what kind of insensitive person would that make me?

Even now, it is very difficult for me to share this with you. These feel like deep, dark secrets that I've hidden for a lifetime that I'm now putting down on paper for the world to see. It's freaky; I'm not going to lie! But hiding them would mean I have something to be ashamed of, and I don't. Fears are natural; we all have them. Not everyone is afraid of emotions, but then again, not everyone is an emotional eater. If I didn't have these fears maybe I wouldn't be one either. That's why I think this is a great first step. Let's identify our fears and then look at them logically and see if we can let them go.

Luckily for you, your answers to this question are completely private. Even so, this is an activity that may make you feel vulnerable and uncomfortable. Take your time doing this; if you need to, take time to digest and reflect on the question for a few days before sitting down to journal about it. Then, create an environment that feels as safe as you can, so that you can feel safe to speak/write your truth. That's paramount—don't sugar coat it; don't minimize your fears; don't avoid writing down and facing the tough stuff. If you truly want to heal and overcome your struggle with emotional eating, you need to face your emotional fears head on. Take a deep breath, and relax. You can do this!

So, let me ask it again. What scares you about feeling or dealing with your emotions?

How do you feel now that you've written that out?

| |
| |
| |
| |
| |
| |

For me, just getting it out of my heart and onto paper gave me a huge sense of relief. As I mentioned earlier, it felt like I had been holding onto deep dark secrets that I was finally able to release.

When you are ready, I want you to re-read what you wrote and look at each fear logically to determine the reality of the situation. For example, I wrote that I am afraid of losing control. What I am really afraid of is physically lashing out at someone I love if I allow myself to feel the full extent of my anger. That's no small concern. However, if I look at reality, there's little probability of that ever happening.

1. I'm 41 years old and I've never hit anyone in my life.
2. I am a future thinker, so even in the heat of the moment I tend to consider future consequences before speaking or lashing out. Physicality is a very present-minded reaction, which isn't a typical part of my M.O.
3. In many ways I am a control freak, so I can't imagine allowing myself to lose so much self-control that I hit someone I care about just because I'm angry.
4. Now that I know that it is a fear, I can watch for it when I explore my feelings of anger and ensure that I control it.

Although I have a fear of losing control, when I look at it logically, there's very little probability I'll actually lose my temper to the point of physically hurting someone. So, I can let go of that fear.

If you are thinking that that is an easy fear to reason out, I agree. So, let's look at a tougher one—my fear of looking/ feeling vulnerable.

Eleanor Roosevelt once said, "No one can make you feel inferior without your consent."

This falls directly in line with my fear. The only way I can feel vulnerable is if I choose to feel vulnerable. Sadness, hurt, frustration, or any of the other many emotions out there cannot make me feel vulnerable unless I allow it. If someone hurts my feelings, I ultimately choose my reaction to that. I can

> The only way I can feel vulnerable is if I choose to feel vulnerable.

choose to feel like a victim and feel sorry for myself. I can choose to be angry and lash out. Or I can choose to assume the other person had a positive intent and investigate why I feel hurt. All of these are choices. Knowing that I can control my feelings of vulnerability helps me to release some of the power that fear has over me.

Using my two examples as a guide, re-read the fears that you wrote on the previous pages, and look at each fear logically to determine the reality of the situation.

The fear:
The logical reality:

The fear:

The logical reality:

The fear:

The logical reality:

The fear:

The logical reality:

Hopefully, this exercise helped you begin to make peace with your fears by realizing that they are either improbable or controllable. If you came across any fears that you weren't able to make peace with, put a star beside them and either find a counselor that can help you, reach out to me so we can talk through it, or find someone you trust who can help you to make peace with that fear.

Figure out how you use food to deal with emotions

There are three primary ways that we use food to deal with emotions: to comfort, to distract, and to punish ourselves. Most emotional eaters know that they use food for both comfort and distraction. Most likely it is something we learned from our parents when we were growing up. It's not their fault; they learned it from *their* parents too. Unfortunately, this taught us two lessons: 1) It isn't okay to feel unhappy, so if you feel unhappy, get yourself back to feeling happy as fast as possible, and 2) food can help us to get there.

We brought these lessons with us into adulthood, and now we constantly avoid feeling unhappy, and when we become unhappy, we immediately turn to food to get back to happy. We have no desire to face or feel our emotions, so we distract ourselves with food. As long as we are busy concentrating on food, we can't concentrate on the hurt, anger, sadness, dissatisfaction, etc. that we feel. This allows us to ignore our emotions in the hopes that they will go away and we will never have to deal with them.

If distraction isn't enough and an emotion does sneak through, food becomes a comfort instead of a distraction. When we are focused on the present moment and aren't looking towards the future, it seems as if food can't hurt us. It doesn't talk back, it doesn't turn its back on us, it doesn't say mean things, it doesn't lash out in anger. Instead, food looks, smells, feels, and tastes delicious, which brings us pleasure at a moment when we are feeling anything but happy. It's no wonder we turn to food when we feel badly! Unfortunately, using food for comfort typically means eating too much of a food that is high in fat, flour, or sugar, which leads us into the binge/guilt/binge cycle.

It's important that we stop this cycle, both for ourselves and for our children. If you are a parent, one of the best things you can do for your children is to break this unhealthy pattern and begin a new, healthier one. When your child comes to you upset, simply hold them and let them cry. Listen without judgment as they explain what's wrong. Encourage them to talk to whoever upset them. If it was some*thing* rather than some*one* that upset them, let them explore why it upset them and encourage them to think about what they can do to resolve the issue. Don't rush them out of their unhappiness, and DON'T OFFER THEM FOOD! Obviously, this is a good practice to use on yourself, as well, but you've already been trained differently, so it may be a bit tougher than that. We'll get to that in a few pages. ☺

Let's talk about another way we use food, which probably caught your attention and curiosity earlier. This may surprise a lot of you, but many of us use food to subconsciously punish ourselves. Have you ever been in a situation where you swore to yourself, over and over again, that you would be strong and wouldn't eat that brownie? However, five minutes later it was down your throat and settled in your belly before you even knew what you were doing? Then you started to berate yourself for being weak and said, "Screw it! I've already screwed up my diet so I might as well eat the rest." That, my friend, is punishment. Basically, you are subconsciously thinking a version of, "I am weak-willed and will obviously never achieve my goal. I don't deserve to lose weight because I'm fat and weak, with no self-control, so here you go fatty—stuff your gullet. That's what you want to do anyway!" Between the negative self-talk and gorging on "bad" food, we punish ourselves for being "bad." Does that sound familiar? Tell me that isn't the most negative scenario we can create for ourselves!?

It doesn't just happen when we deviate from our diet plan and eat something "bad." It can happen anytime we feel guilt. Think about the last time you lashed out or wronged a loved one. When your emotions calmed down, you most likely felt guilty about your behavior. What did you do next? How did you deal with it?

Guilt is a very strong emotion, and it makes us feel badly about ourselves and whatever it is we did or said. No one likes to feel guilty, and many of us don't like to admit that we were wrong and apologize. The act of saying "I'm sorry, I was wrong" is the appropriate "punishment" that would actually allow the wronged person to forgive us, as well as allowing us to forgive ourselves. But, if we avoid apologizing, we continue to carry the guilt with us. This may sound weird, but when we do that, we crave punishment to atone for whatever it is that caused the guilt in the first place. I've found that the primary ways an emotional eater self-punishes is through negative self-talk and gorging on "bad" food to perpetuate our self-disgust.

If this concept makes you uncomfortable, angry, or immediately resistant, stop and journal. Remember, when we feel our greatest discomfort or resistance, we are actually onto something that's vitally important to our journey to health. Determine what it is about this theory that makes you uncomfortable or upset. Continue to journal or think about it until you come up with your conclusions.

Even if you aren't resistant to the idea of food as punishment, journal about your overall thoughts on how and/or why you use food for comfort, distraction, and punishment.

Figure out what you are actually feeling when you want to reach for food

The process of *experiencing* emotions in a healthy manner is very similar to a wave in the ocean. The emotions build and grow momentum until they can't build anymore, then they crash, calm and retreat. As long as you allow your emotions to crash, meaning as long as you are willing to feel and experience them, then they will calm and retreat. The process of *suppressing* emotions is very similar to a shaken can of soda. As you continue to avoid, distract, or suppress your emotions, they just build and build and build, adding more and more pressure without the ability to release it. That will either cause small leaks, making you irritable and short tempered without any obvious cause, or it will cause a huge explosion where you emotionally and destructively spew all of the suppressed emotion you've been bottling up all over everyone around you.

Needless to say, we need to start transitioning our behaviors from that of a shaken can of soda to that of a wave. To do that, we need to recognize how each of our emotions manifests itself, and then determine the best way of experiencing the emotion so we can let it run its course and then let it go.

> As long as you are willing to feel and experience your emotions, they will calm and retreat.

You may be so out of touch with your emotions that you may not even know what your emotions feel like. In that case, a good exercise is for you to describe what you think sadness, hurt, anger, disappointment, frustration, etc. would feel like to you physically, mentally and emotionally. For example, I used to fiercely suppress any feelings of hurt and pretend that people couldn't hurt me. Well, we all know that as a human, we can be hurt by someone. So, I went through this exercise and learned what I should look for physically, mentally and emotionally so I can recognize when I feel hurt.

Physically, when I feel hurt, I feel a heaviness or a pressure in my chest. I feel a strong need to cry. I start to shake, and I feel like I want to crawl out of my skin. Mentally, I want to go into hiding. I want to isolate myself and keep everyone and everything away from me. I completely shut down and retract into myself like a turtle. Emotionally, I tend to run through a continuous cycle of feeling defensive, angry, rejected and dejected. Of all these reactions, the need to isolate myself from others is the strongest sign that tells me I've been hurt. Once I identify that I want to run and hide from the world, I know I'm feeling hurt. That's my indicator or "tell" that I am feeling a strong emotion that I need to let out and explore. At that point, I force myself to stop and journal about the situation until I can identify the cause of the hurt, why that specifically hurt me, and how I can resolve it so that the hurt can recede. This allows my emotion to build, have its crescendo, and then melt away.

So, if you aren't sure what your various emotions feel like, run through this exercise to figure out what your "tell" is for each emotion. Once you know your tells, you can stop your forward momentum and actually let your emotions run their course.

Emotion:		
Physical Manifestation	**Mental Manifestation**	**Emotional Manifestation**

Emotion:		
Physical Manifestation	**Mental Manifestation**	**Emotional Manifestation**

Figure out what your "tells" are for each emotion
so you can stop your forward momentum
and let your emotions run their course.

Emotion:		
Physical Manifestation	**Mental Manifestation**	**Emotional Manifestation**

Emotion:		
Physical Manifestation	**Mental Manifestation**	**Emotional Manifestation**

Once you have determined what your tells are for each emotion, it is vital that when you experience a tell you stop, explore the feeling, and allow yourself to experience the sadness, anger, frustration, hurt, etc. At first, simply focus on identifying what emotion you are feeling. Once you can do that consistently, determine what you need to do to release that emotion. Find a healthy outlet for both experiencing and letting go of the emotion. For some people, like me, the best outlet is journaling; for others it is working through the situation in their minds while going for a walk. Or, maybe crying works best for you. Don't be afraid to cry. Meditating on the cause of the emotion and releasing it during yoga, or punching a punching bag are also great ways to release emotion. Venting to a friend or confidante is another great option. These are only a few examples of the many outlets you can use to explore your emotions. What is important is finding the best outlet for *you*, one that allows you time to digest and work through what you are feeling so you can release it without using food.

> Find a healthy outlet that lets you experience and let go of the emotion.

Figure out what would comfort you in the situation that caused the emotion, without using food

A few years ago, I was hurt by someone I considered to be a friend. Out of the blue, the person accused me of acting out of disrespect and cut off our friendship. It was a shock, to say the least, and it broke my heart that a "friend" would trust me so little and accuse me so quickly of something I would never do—and all through a text. At the time I read the text, I immediately began to shake, my chest filled with pressure, and I felt the need to run and hide. Whoa! Those were obvious tells that I was really feeling hurt. At the time, I was in the midst of working with back-to-back clients, so I had no chance to deal with the hurt, but luckily, I also didn't have time to eat.

When I *did* have time, I immediately grabbed my laptop and began to journal. I was able to figure out what it was about the situation that hurt me. I was able to write out all of the hurt until I felt empty. At which point, I realized that my "friend" was lashing out as a result of her own insecurity. Her insecurity caused her to lash out at me, unfairly, because she was incapable of being logical rather than emotional. She had the opposite problem to mine; she felt her emotions so strongly that she couldn't control them. Once I realized that the situation had nothing to do with my actions and everything to do with her insecurity, I got really angry at the injustice of it! So, I then journaled about my anger and eventually wrote a response to her text. I never sent the response to her, but just by clearly writing out the reality of the situation and standing up for myself, even just in my journal, I felt vindicated, relieved of any guilt she tried to make me feel, and back in control. Once I was able to calm my emotions of hurt and anger, I was able to let them go, which negated my need for food as comfort.

That is just one example of how I use journaling to comfort me when I feel strong emotions. There are no expectations when I journal. I don't have to be logical, or fair, or reasonable; I don't have to spell correctly or use good grammar. I don't have to write in a way that is easy for others to follow; I don't have to monitor my language; I don't have to answer any questions, solve any problems or do anything other than write whatever I feel like writing at the time. It doesn't even need to make sense.

That's why journaling is a great outlet for me. There are no rules about how to do it, and I can write whatever I need to in order to calm my chaotic mind, figure out what I'm feeling, and what I should do about it. Journaling is very freeing for me. I also know that once I feel back in control, my true comfort comes from talking about it with people I trust to love me through thick and thin. These people say the things I want and need to hear during my emotional turmoil. They will listen, give me a hug if I need it, and rally in my corner. Between journaling and then venting to people that I trust to love me, I get the comfort I need to stay away from food.

Think about what would comfort you in the midst of feeling strong emotions and write it below. If you aren't sure, then brainstorm a few options and see what resonates with you.

As Brené Brown has proven through her research, there's nothing as fulfilling and uplifting as love and connection, and we cannot experience those to the fullest unless we also experience sadness and hurt. Hopefully, this knowledge will give you the impetus you need to forge ahead through your fear and continue to work on acknowledging, experiencing and releasing your emotions. Although it feels scary and vulnerable to really feel our emotions, the rewards of forging onward are epic. And, although we have been turning to food for comfort for many, many years, working through these exercises can help you to break this habit and make feeling your emotions less scary.

CHAPTER 10

Take Away Food's Power

Now that we've committed to feeling our emotions, it's time to put food in its place. Food is meant to nourish our bodies so we can feel and do our best in life. That's it. It isn't meant to be a reward, a mode of celebration, a distraction from boredom, a comfort from sadness, or any of the other myriad roles we give it; it is meant to nourish our bodies. When we give food all of these other roles and responsibilities, it is constantly front and center in our lives and we can't get away from it. That gives food way too much power and stage-time in our lives that it just doesn't deserve. Just think, life is always providing us with reasons to celebrate, distract ourselves, avoid something, or need comfort, so if we depend on food to get us through each of those situations we will constantly be eating—which is the very habit we need to change.

So, let's talk about finding alternatives to food for these various situations in our lives so food can do what we need it to do: nourish our bodies.

Let's start by determining the primary areas in our lives in which we turn to food. I primarily turn to food when I:

1. Am bored
2. Am pissed off
3. Am stressed

4. Want to socialize
5. Want to procrastinate
6. Want to celebrate/reward myself
7. Want to punish myself

What about you? Take a moment and list the various situations in which you turn to food.

Now that we know when we give food a role it doesn't deserve, let's find some alternatives to food that we can turn to instead. Let's use boredom, from my list, as an example.

Here is a list I keep handy of things I can do instead of eating when I'm bored:

- Look at cool new posts on Pinterest
- Call and catch up with a friend
- Catch up with friends on Facebook
- Go for a hike (I have a mountain practically in my backyard!)
- Read up on creative new exercises or recipes
- Go take an exercise class or workout at the gym

- Clean my house (I never choose this option...go figure!)
- Go to the store and buy myself a new book
- Go to the grocery store and check out what's new in the health food section (yep, I'm a nerd ☺)
- Try out a new recipe (I love cooking! And I typically don't eat when I cook. Weird, I know!)
- Write another chapter in my book (obviously this one is no longer on my list...if you have any good book ideas for me, maybe I can add this one back on my list ☺)
- Journal
- Give myself a facial
- Give myself a pedicure
- Window shop on the internet (this requires self-control, so be careful with this one ☺)
- Take a nap

The important part of this list is to incorporate things you would actually enjoy doing. The simple truth is, we really enjoy eating so we need something else that's just as enticing to do as an alternative. You've probably heard people advise that you go for a walk when you are bored, but if I had a choice between eating Ben and Jerry's or going for a walk, guess which one has more allure? However, I am a total nerd and really enjoy reading labels at the grocery store. I could do that for hours. In fact, I've spent many a Friday night in the grocery store checking out new foods in the health food section and reading the labels. I also love cooking and trying out new recipes. Since I cook in bulk and eat 90% of my meals reheated, I don't feel the compulsion to eat what I cook, so I can make something delicious and then pack it away to eat later. I also love Zumba, playing with our dog, exploring the desert, and catching up with friends. These are things I truly enjoy, so it makes it easy to replace eating with those activities.

Pick the first item from your list above and think about realistic and enjoyable alternatives to eating in that scenario.

Scenario:

| |
| |
| |
| Alternatives: |
| |
| |
| |
| |

Continue with this activity for each of the scenarios on your list until you have a good list of alternatives for each of them.

Scenario:

| |
| |
| |
| Alternatives: |
| |
| |
| |
| |

Scenario:

Alternatives:

Scenario:

Alternatives:

Scenario:

Alternatives:

Scenario:

Alternatives:

Scenario:

Alternatives:

Now, what are you going to do with these lists?

I hang mine on the refrigerator. It is a great reminder to take stock and determine whether I'm actually hungry or turning to food for other reasons before I open the fridge and start eating. It also reminds me about all of my alternatives if I'm not really hungry.

As I've mentioned frequently throughout this book, be patient with yourself as you develop new habits. This is a journey; you aren't going to go from emotional eating to NOT emotionally eating overnight. Start by paying attention when you get the urge to eat. If you shouldn't feel hungry because you ate within the last few hours, then most likely something else is contributing to your feelings of hunger. At that point, figure out what it is before taking the first bite. Then, go to your lists, find an alternative activity and do that instead.

The key is to actually start replacing food with the activities on your lists as soon as possible; your lists are only as helpful as the action you take from them.

CHAPTER 11

Triggers

As we continue to pay attention to our eating habits around feelings and food, we will learn more and more about the many ways that food has controlled our lives. You may find that despite adopting the various techniques we have discussed in this book, there will still be times when you feel out of control around food. There may be specific emotions, situations or foods that cause a loss of control and set off a binge; these are called triggers.

I have quite a few of them. Boredom. Excitement. Stress. Social settings. Celebrations. Eating out. Skipping meals. Dark Chocolate. Dessert. Organics Teddy Grahams. Stacey's Pita Chips. Cheese. Pasta. Bread. Tortilla chips.

These are my triggers. Probably not all of them, but these are definitely the major ones that come to mind when I think about it. Notice that there are feelings, situations, *and* foods that act as triggers. I'm not immune to triggers, even after all of these years. Despite my greater ability to feel, express, and release my emotions, there are still times when I fall into a binge and find myself stuffed and feeling out of control. The good news is that my binges happen much less frequently. I still have my emotional challenges with food, but I've found methods that allow me to win the binging war most of the time. Yay, me! Good girl! ☺

So, what are my methods of coping with my triggers? They aren't the same for each trigger, and they may not work for you, just as you may have your own triggers that don't match mine.

A great first step is identifying what your triggers are, similar to what I did above. Since this is a book about emotional eating, let's start with emotions. My primary emotional triggers are happiness and stress. Some of you would argue that stress isn't an emotion, but a lot of my stress comes from what goes on in my head, so for me, stress is an emotion. And really, who cares? It needs to go on a trigger list, so as long as it makes it on one, who cares where I put it, right? So, in that same vein, don't overanalyze what trigger should be listed on which list. This is your journey, so you get to put whatever you want on your list, wherever you want it ☺. Take a few minutes and do some soul searching. Figure out which emotions cause you to turn to food for comfort, distraction or punishment.

My Emotional Triggers

| |
| |
| |
| |
| |
| |
| |

Now, let's look at *situations* that act as triggers. Social settings are the worst for me. I am an extrovert that enjoys getting together with friends, and yet I don't get the opportunity to do that too often. So, when I have the chance to socialize (trigger) I get super excited (trigger) and want to celebrate (trigger). It's a triple whammy! Then, because food and alcohol are typically at the center of every social event, I am surrounded by temptation—the kind of temptation I typically avoid in my day-to-day life. So, not only do I have a variety of triggers going off that sabotage my self-control, but I am surrounded by all of the unhealthy foods that I crave and rarely allow myself to eat. For me, this can be a recipe for disaster.

What situations do you run into that trigger your desire to binge?

My Situational Triggers

Now, let's focus on food. There are certain foods that trigger a binge, or at least the desire to binge. You know, those foods that if you have an entire bag/box/bowl/plate in front of you, you'll eat the entire thing and then still want more. Yup, those foods.

Kettle corn!

Sorry, that was random, but as we sit here discussing trigger foods, another one of mine came to mind. I can't seem to stop eating kettle corn once I start, so that goes on the list.

Anyway, trigger foods are very similar to cocaine, to me. They give us a quick high followed by a heavy crash, and they are addictive and destructive both mentally and physically.

Take a moment and think of the various foods that trigger your binge reflex and list them here. Just to be clear, this is not a list of foods you crave. This is a list of the foods you cannot stop eating once you start.

My Food Triggers

As I mentioned earlier and demonstrated above, you'll probably come up with more triggers as you have more time to think about it. No biggie, just add them to your list as they pop into your head.

Identifying your triggers is a great first step, although I bet most of you are already aware of what your triggers are. However, having them in writing takes that awareness to another level.

Now that you know what your triggers are, you can come up with a plan for overcoming them. Everybody uses different methods; finding the right methods for you will require some soul searching. In fact, you may benefit from re-reading Chapter 3 and using some of those activities to determine what actions you are willing to take to avoid triggering your...ahem...triggers.

For example, I LOVE, LOVE, LOVE dark chocolate and so far, I have been unwilling to give it up on a forever basis. However, when I feel as if I am losing control over my cravings, I will completely remove it from my life for a month or two to hit my reset button. That seems to work for me. It's a great way to live in my gray world, rather than cutting it out of my life entirely.

Another example is eating out. I LOVE, LOVE, LOVE to eat out. I love the sights and the smells and the atmosphere when I eat out. I love trying new foods and flavors I've never had before. I love eating a freshly cooked meal prepared by someone else. I love walking away from the dirty dishes when I'm done. There isn't a single thing about eating out I don't like except for maybe the bill. But, because the food is so yummy—and served in such large portions—I struggle not to binge in that setting. Luckily, I have an amazing man in my life who understands my struggles, is willing to be a great support system for me, and is willing to take control. Also, my desire to be healthy supersedes my need to be independent, so I'm willing to give up control in that situation. When we eat out, my boyfriend does me the favor of ordering for me. He knows what I enjoy and has a good understanding of the balance between delicious and nutritious, so he will pick something from the menu that I can enjoy and feel good about eating. It takes all of the pressure off of me to make the best choice. Then, because portion control is a big issue for me, he does a great job of lovingly suggesting when I've had enough. He has a gift for doing that without causing me to feel patronized, judged, or belittled. In all honesty, it makes me feel supported and loved. He's looking out for my best interests when I'm at my weakest. Instead of being resentful, I'm grateful.

Some people would not be willing to give up that level of control to someone else, so this method would not be an option for them, but it shows that there are a variety of unorthodox methods out there, if you are willing to live in the gray and be creative. So, let's work on coming up with some methods, creative or otherwise, that may work for you.

Notice that I used the word "may." Some of this process is trial and error. If an idea resonates with you, try it and see if it works for you. If not, then don't hesitate to adapt it, or get rid of it and try something else. This is a journey, so expect some detours as you find the best path to take. ☺

Since the first list we created cataloged our emotional triggers, let's start there. In the last chapter, you learned the importance of allowing yourself to feel and experience all of your emotions. You came up with techniques for exploring emotions you had avoided feeling in the past. As you have learned, allowing yourself to feel and experience your most challenging emotions reduces their power over you and stops the trigger reaction of overeating. For most emotional triggers, experiencing the emotion head-on is enough to stave off a binge reaction. However, you may need some additional techniques ready to use to avoid a binge.

For example, I typically feel stressed when I am overwhelmed with too much to do and too little time, or when I have a lot of tasks on my to-do list I'd rather avoid than do. In those instances, simply embracing the feeling of being stressed is not helpful.

Instead, I have found a few different techniques that help me. First, I stop and write down everything I have to get done so it is no longer clogging up my brain. Next, I determine when each task needs to be done, realistically. Then, based on the tasks I want to avoid, I either treat them like medicine and do them all at once in one fell swoop to get them over with, or I spread them out so I am not stuck doing a whole bunch of things I hate at once.

For me, having a plan calms me down and takes me from being emotional to being logical. It immediately squelches my desire to binge because I feel back in control.

Take a few minutes to think through which emotional triggers are strong enough that you may need some additional techniques besides experiencing the emotion. Come up with some possible techniques that could help you to stave off an eating binge.

Emotional Trigger:

Techniques for avoiding an emotional binge when triggered:

Emotional Trigger:

Techniques for avoiding an emotional binge when triggered:

Emotional Trigger:

Techniques for avoiding an emotional binge when triggered:

Emotional Trigger:

Techniques for avoiding an emotional binge when triggered:

Situational triggers are next. For each of your situational triggers, I want you to:

1. Identify below what it is about each situation that causes the trigger.
2. Brainstorm various things you can do to set yourself up to avoid a binge in that situation. This is a brainstorm, so your options don't need to be realistic or appealing, simply possible options. Also, don't just rely on your own brain for creative ideas. Do an internet search, read other books on emotional eating, talk to other emotional eaters, etc. You aren't alone, so don't isolate yourself. Use all of your resources to come up with possible techniques. Just because a technique is on this list doesn't mean you are going to adopt it.
3. Determine which actions on your list you *are* willing to adopt.

Situational Trigger

What about this situation causes the trigger?

Brainstorm ways to avoid the binge:

List the actions you *are* willing to try:

Situational Trigger

What about this situation causes the trigger?

Brainstorm ways to avoid the binge:

List the actions you *are* willing to try:

Situational Trigger

What about this situation causes the trigger?

Brainstorm ways to avoid the binge:

List the actions you are *willing* to try:

Situational Trigger

What about this situation causes the trigger?

Brainstorm ways to avoid the binge:

List the actions you are *willing* to try:

As I mentioned earlier, trigger foods can create an addictive reaction in the body very similar to cocaine. You know that you are addicted if you physically cannot stop yourself from gorging on a food or drink once you've had a taste of it. If that is the case, I suggest doing some serious soul searching over the idea of removing trigger foods from your diet entirely. This has nothing to do with weight loss and everything to do with addiction recovery. With any addictive substance, there is no such thing as a taste. Addictive substances cause a chemical change in the brain that is out of your control. What you *do* control is whether you ingest the addictive substance in the first place. Even if you don't suffer from an actual addiction to your trigger foods, they are still triggers that either cause you to overeat or feel guilt after eating them. Even without an addiction I would consider removing them from your diet, at least temporarily.

The thought of removing your favorite foods may seem daunting, so this is a good time to stop and journal. Here are some things you may want to explore while you are journaling:

- What was your initial reaction when you read that you should remove your trigger foods entirely from your diet?
- If you feel a tremendous amount of resistance to the idea of removing these foods entirely from your diet, explore why. Then, complete the change process activity in Chapter 3 and explore what you *are* willing to do.

If you feel a lot of resistance and resentment towards this topic, allow yourself a few days to work through this journaling exercise. You'll get more out of it if you allow yourself time to digest and reflect, rather than trying to push your way through it all at once.

Did you have any revelations?

When we feel the greatest amount of resistance, we are usually on the brink of a great discovery—if we simply allow ourselves time to reflect and work through it. In the past, you may have avoided this type of challenge and simply ate or even binged instead. Now, you are facing your challenges and working through them, rather than eating. That's a really big success!

So, as you can see from the previous activities, triggers can take many forms and can have varying degrees of severity. The tricks to controlling your reaction to triggers are:

1. identifying what your triggers are.
2. minimizing your exposure to triggers (ideally *avoiding* addictive triggers).
3. creating effective action plans for your most common triggers.
4. recognizing when you're being triggered.
5. implementing your action plan as soon as possible.

Preparation is the name of the game. By walking into any given situation, emotion, or food with awareness and an action plan, your odds of handling any possible triggers successfully are exponentially higher. With continued success, and consistent use of your "praise phrase," food will have less control over you. Then, your confidence and feeling of self-worth will skyrocket, until you are the confident, successful, happy person you deserve to be.

CHAPTER 12

Reduce Stress

As I mentioned in the last chapter, stress is one of my triggers, and suspect it is for many of you, as well. We are our own worst enemy, and when it comes to stress there are no truer words. There are some stresses we just can't get away from, but there are probably just as many that we can, and yet we continue to allow stress into our lives. Stress reduces our ability to focus on ourselves and on our needs. It steals the energy and passion we need to enjoy our lives, enjoy our food, feel our emotions, and connect with other people—all of which brings us the fulfillment we need so we don't feel compelled to emotionally eat.

Although there are a ton of books, coaches, articles, and videos on the various techniques we can use to better *handle* stress, I want to challenge you to actually *reduce* your stress. I want you to take a very honest look at your life and determine what stressors you can remove. I don't want you to think about how you can handle your various stressors better; I want you to remove them.

Here's an example. I started writing this book more than three years ago, when my client base was a lot smaller. I was able to focus almost entirely on the book and had the energy and passion to allow the words to flow. Writing the book was a pleasure; it was invigorating, fulfilling and free-flowing. I had the time, energy and inspiration for the suggestions that I wanted to share, and they flowed freely onto the paper. Then, my business took off and my client base doubled, practically overnight. All of a sudden, I went from working 10-20 hours per week to working 10-12 hours per day. Yikes! There went all of my time, energy and creativity for writing this book.

Here was something that I was so excited about, something that inspired me and hopefully would inspire and help others, and all of a sudden it became a stressor instead of a joy. It was no longer something I was creating to help and inspire others; instead, it turned into an obligation, something else for me to do. That is the last thing I wanted this book to be. There was no way I could create the inspiration I wanted for others if I was simply writing out of obligation. So, I tabled it. I put it aside and took it off of my list of things to do until I could refocus on it with the proper energy and attention that would allow me to enjoy the process rather than stress out about simply getting it done.

If I had only focused on getting this book finished, it would not have had the same impact on you as it does now. By taking my time and shelving it until it was a better time for *me*, I could write the book I always wanted to publish—one written from my heart. If I had allowed it to become an obligation, it would have ended up flat and dry. Did my plans for my business have to wait? Yes. Was I often questioned about my progress on the book? You know it! Did it hurt my pride to have to tell my friends, family and clients that I hadn't made any progress on it in over a year? You betcha! But, you know what? Once I gave myself permission to shelve the book until I had the time and energy to devote to it, I immediately felt a sense of relief. The only true deadline was the one I set for myself. What was the consequence of not hitting my deadline? I wouldn't be able to start my emotional eaters program as soon as I wanted to. Well, you know what? I was too busy anyway! I didn't have a single slot in my schedule to hold the meetings I wanted to pair with this book. So, putting myself into a tizzy to finish something because I made an arbitrary deadline, or because my pride was hurt to admit I wasn't done with it yet would have been senseless. So, I gave myself kudos every day for being wise enough to table writing the book until the right time.

Now, I want to challenge you to do the same thing. I'm not going to lie; this is going to be a challenge because we feel such an obligation to do and do and do, but you can't dedicate the time and energy you need to yourself if you continue to give it away to everyone and everything else.

To steal a question from Erin Ramsey's book, *Be Amazing*, "What makes us think that we can perform wonderfully and give freely if we are exhausted and don't even know what we have on hand to give?"

I want you to take the next 20-30 minutes and list *everything* in your life that causes you stress. Don't worry about judgment; don't worry about what other people will think—no one else is going to read this—and don't worry about being too detailed. I want you to write out all the stresses in your life, big and small, and I don't want you to move on with this chapter until you've completed this activity. I want you to list all of the ways that your spouse/partner, your kids, your job, your boss, your mother, father, etc. add stress to your life. You aren't going to hurt anyone's feelings; this is simply the truth— *your* truth! Write your list and make it all-encompassing.

What causes stress in my life?

You are not done yet.

Now, I want you to go back and re-read each item on your list and ask yourself the following questions after you read each item.

"What would be the consequence(s) if I stopped doing that?" "What's the worst that could happen?"

"What's the best that could happen?"

"Could I live with the worst?"

Even if only 75% of your heart can accept the worst that could happen, that's enough—cross it off your list.

This is not a comfortable exercise, so you aren't going to be all hunky-dory to drop tasks or activities you've felt obligated to complete for the last few months or years. It's okay to feel uncomfortable in this process. Remember, we are embracing our emotions and allowing ourselves to feel and explore them as they come up. If you are very uncomfortable after this exercise, I want you to stop and journal. Work through whatever is uncomfortable so that you can embrace this idea of letting go of stress in your life.

What is causing me stress and why am I uncomfortable about giving it up?

What's the worst that could happen?

What's the best that could happen?

By the time you are finished asking those questions, you should have cut your list of obligations down by at least 25%. If you haven't, I recommend putting this book aside for now, and coming back to the exercise tomorrow or the next day and trying again because this is crucial. Reducing the number of stressors in your life is the difference between having time and not having time. It is the difference between having energy and not having energy. It is the difference between enjoying your life and simply working through your life. It is the difference between having the ability to take care of yourself or continuing your habit of taking care of everyone and everything else—to your own detriment.

Which brings us to the next exercise. Go back through the items that you have left on your list and ask, "Who else can do this besides me?" You are not the only capable person in your life. Others may not do the job the way you would, or exactly to your standards, but they can do it! Your way isn't the only way. And if your standards are keeping you from delegating, then you are once again being your own worst enemy; you are making the choice to give your time and energy away rather than taking care of yourself. Is it really worth that?

When I ask clients who they can delegate tasks to, their number one response is, "Oh, but I can't ask so-and-so because they are just too busy!" You know what my response is? "So are you! Why is their time more valuable than yours?" The truth is, theirs isn't. You simply don't value yourself the way you should.

So, with this in mind, go back through your list and ask yourself, "Who else can do this besides me?" Don't worry about anyone else's time, simply worry about their knowledge and ability to do the task currently on your list. And be honest about your spouse and kids. They are way more capable than you give them credit for. Delegate!

Whew...we are almost done! The last thing to do is to delegate the various tasks to the people you have determined can do them. Yes, I know. I know! This is uncomfortable and everyone else is busy too! But, so are you, and you are finally ready to take care of yourself, remember? That's why you bought this book. This is part of it. Fighting for yourself, your time and your energy is part of the process of developing a healthier lifestyle without emotional eating. You will know that you finally matter when you begin to fight for yourself. And if you aren't there yet, fake it 'til you make it. This means that you fight for yourself even if you aren't yet convinced you are worth it; fight for yourself even though it is uncomfortable and you don't want to do it. You can't make a new habit until the old habit is broken. Consider it a test...one you want to pass for the betterment of your psyche, the betterment of your family, the betterment of your career, and the betterment of your life.

Here's some motivation.

If you were to get rid of at least 25% of the tasks on your list, how much time would that open up for you?

How could you use that time on your journey to overcome emotional eating and challenges with weight loss? How could you use that time to fulfill your emotional needs?

Example: Read
Example: Journal
Example: Prepare, cook, and pack my meals for the week.
Example: Spend time with my family, friends, significant other
Example: Have some quiet time for myself

How could you use that time to better enjoy your life? Dream! Create your new reality!

Example: Finally learn how to play golf.
Example: Finally take that weekend trip.

Your new reality will become a possibility when you have the time and energy to create it. So, don't make this a thought experiment. Own it, and start removing the unnecessary stressors from your life... today!

CHAPTER 13

Support System

Since we talked about eliminating and reducing stress in the last chapter, let's talk about another way we can make this journey of overcoming emotional eating less stressful: by creating a support system. You've heard me mention my amazing boyfriend a few times in this book. He is one of my major support systems and without him my successes wouldn't be nearly as consistent. Studies prove that people going through substantial changes in their life are significantly more successful when they have a strong support system. And it's much more fun! Think about it; have you ever gone on a really long road trip alone? BOOOOORRRRRIIIINNNGG! Now, add a couple of friends on the trip and that long drive turns into a blast! There is no reason you should have to travel alone on your journey to freedom from emotional eating, especially since it is a lifetime journey.

So, let's start by defining what I mean by a "support system." My definition of a support system is the people that I spend the most time with or who play the biggest role in my life helping me to succeed. For example, I spend the most time with my boyfriend, his kids, my oldest brother and his wife, my clients and my girlfriends. They make up a big part of my support system. Then, there are those people that live too far away for me to spend much time with, but who still have a big impact on my life. My mom is a great example! She is also an emotional eater and she understands my journey, so although we are across the country from each other, we talk on the phone frequently and I know I can always count on her to provide unconditional support when I need it.

Think about who you spend the most time with, as well as those that impact your life the most and make a list of who belongs in your support system? This list should only include people that you feel safe with and trust. Don't forget to add your children on the list, if that applies.

That was the easy part. Now, it's time to soul search again.

We've all heard the adage, "Beauty is in the eyes of the beholder." So is the definition of support. I may define support very differently than you; it's not fair to expect your friends to automatically understand what you need them to do to support you. It is human nature for each person to come at a situation from their own point of view; it's the only view they have. As such, if you ask for my support, I will be more than happy to give it to you! The problem is, I'm going to give you *my* version of support, not necessarily the kind of support you want from me.

A friend and I were working out the other day and got onto the topic of how sorry we feel for our men when they try to support us and we reject it. This got us talking further about what works and doesn't work for each of us. I explained how David will order meals in a restaurant for me and then move the plate aside when I've had enough to eat, and how that works really well for me. My friend laughed and said there was no way she'd allow her husband to do that; it would only piss her off, which would make her want to eat more. However, what worked for her was for him to smack her hand whenever she reached for anything she shouldn't be eating. It was my turn to laugh, because that would just make me want to smack David back! Ha ha! We obviously have very different definitions of support, and I would bet dollars to donuts that most men would hesitate to take a woman's plate away or smack her hand without being told to do so first, for fear of her wrath. That's what I mean by not forcing your

> Your Ideal
> Support System:
> - Create *your* definition of support
> - Identify who belongs in your support system
> - Determine what you need from each supporter
> - Clearly communicate your need

support system to guess what your needs are. You've got to clearly define what your version of support is and what you specifically need from them so that they can truly support you, *your* way.

This leads to my first soul searching question of the chapter. Do you know what your version of support is? Do you know what your loved ones can do to support you that will make you feel loved and supported rather than judged and defensive? Do you know how your expectations/needs will differ for each person in your support group?

If you do, awesome! Outline it here so that it is nice and clear.

| |
| |
| |
| |
| |
| |
| |
| |

If you don't know how you want each member of your support group to support you, use the space below to brainstorm some options, recognizing that you may want each person in your support system to support you in different ways. Think about what expectations and boundaries need to be set per person or situation. For example, I wouldn't allow anyone else but David to order for me or take my plate away. But I really appreciate it when my sister-in-law stocks the house with healthy food when I'm coming for a visit. She always makes sure that the meals are healthy, and free of both gluten and dairy to meet my needs. That is the perfect way for her to support me when I'm there. As for my brother, he loves his beer and knows I love my vodka but never pressures me to join him in a drink if I'm avoiding alcohol while I'm there. He completely respects my goals and never mentions the fact that I'm drinking bubbly water instead of my favorite mixed drink. That keeps the pressure off, so I can successfully fight any temptations I may feel.

So, keeping in mind that you may want a different version of support from different people, brainstorm what kind of support you want from your support team.

Now that you have an idea of what type of support you want from your support system, it is time to communicate it to them. For some of you this will be no problem. For others, you are starting to feel anxiety just thinking about it.

Before having the conversation with the different members of your support system, think through what you want or need them to know. You don't need to divulge all of the details of this journey if that makes you uncomfortable. You simply need to give them enough information for them to understand how you would like them to help you and why.

Here is an example of what I could say to my brother when I go to visit him on non-drinking weekends:

> Hey bro-face (yes, that's what I call him ☺), I'm avoiding alcohol again this weekend. It would be too easy to drown my stressors from the week, so I think I'm better off without it. So, instead of offering me a vodka tonic when you grab a beer, do you mind just grabbing me one of my bubbly waters from the fridge instead? That'll help me stay on track and avoid temptation. I would really appreciate it!

I think that is nice and simple and to the point. My brother really doesn't need to know that I'm an emotional eater who is trying to gain control over that bad habit and alcohol is part of that bad habit. He doesn't need to know I'm on this lifelong journey and this is a request I will often make. He doesn't need to know it's not just alcohol I'm avoiding but also any other foods that trigger binging. He doesn't need to know any of that. If I feel the need to share that information with him, he'd be all supportive ears, but it isn't necessary in my request for help. So, don't feel obligated to share information you don't want to share simply because you are asking for support.

Here is a little formula for putting together a simple and effective request for support:

Goal: Give a simple explanation of what you are trying to accomplish so your supporter understands the premise for the request, such as "I'm avoiding alcohol again this weekend."

What you need: This is where you define the specifics of the support you want them to give you, such as "Instead of offering me vodka tonic, grab me bubbly water instead."

How it will help you: People intrinsically want to help the people that they like/love. For your supporter, knowing that they will be helping you in some small way is rewarding. Ex: "By grabbing me water instead of vodka, you will help me stay on track and avoid temptation."

Appreciation: Thank them in advance for being willing to support you. "I would really appreciate it!"

Okay, now it's your turn. Think of someone in your support group that you should have a conversation with. Come up with what you can say to them when you request their support.

<table>
<tr><td></td></tr>
<tr><td></td></tr>
<tr><td></td></tr>
<tr><td></td></tr>
<tr><td></td></tr>
<tr><td></td></tr>
<tr><td></td></tr>
<tr><td></td></tr>
</table>

If it will help you, complete this exercise for each person you need to talk to.

Now, let's take a moment to focus on children. Many of you are parents and it would be a big mistake to leave your kids out of this equation. I don't care how old they are. Children have a very large impact on emotional eating habits and need to be brought into your support group so they can contribute to your success rather than your problem. As much as we love our children, they create a lot of stress and mess in our lives. The greater the stress and mess the more we will eat emotionally, which means we need to talk to our kids about what we are trying to accomplish and how they can help us. Whether that's asking them to do a better job with their chores or by being willing to try newer and healthier recipes at dinner, it is important that you communicate your needs and hold them accountable for supporting you.

> It is important to communicate your needs to your children and hold them accountable for supporting you.
>
> **You are worth it!**

You are worth it.

Besides, we generally don't give children enough credit; they are strong, smart, capable little beings that are more than able to help you on this journey along with the various adults you include in your support group. By communicating what you need, you will teach your kids a really good habit that will help them to avoid your emotional eating tendencies.

No matter who you include in your support system, ensure that they understand what you need from them so that you can both be successful on this journey.

CHAPTER 14

You Are Perfectly Imperfect

You are worth it. Did you notice I snuck that into the last chapter? When we discussed the importance of communicating your needs to your children and then holding them accountable for upholding their commitment, I mentioned that you are worth it. You are worth taking care of. You are worth asking for and receiving support. You are worth having your needs fulfilled. You are worth fighting for.

How do you feel after reading that?

I would love it if your reaction to that was, "Hell yeah, I am!"

Unfortunately, most emotional eaters suffer from self-disgust, body image issues, and lack of self-worth. As a result, we often cater to everyone but ourselves. When was the last time you did something "selfish"? When was the last time that you thought about what you wanted or needed and made sure that you got it? What if I told you that the only way to be successful at overcoming emotional eating is to have self-care, a.k.a. "selfish" moments on a consistent basis so that you feel loved first and foremost by yourself?

I know you've heard this before, but the simple truth is that you can't feel or receive love from others unless you love yourself. If you don't love yourself, you don't allow others to show love to you, and you don't allow others to help you or cater to you. If you don't allow others to do things for you, then they won't. People will only accept rejection so often before they give up. Let your friends help you.

Let other parents take charge of the carpool. Let your spouse make the lunches. Let your spouse clean something or cook dinner. You don't have to do it all. Your worth is not in what you do but in who you are.

Emotional eaters often don't believe in their own worth, so they are always hustling for approval because they don't approve of themselves. And yet, when we are constantly doing something, we have zero ability to get in touch with our emotions. We don't have the time or the energy to get our thinking aligned with our actions. We have zero ability to take a breath and think about what it is that *we* need. We are too busy doing, and doing doesn't allow for thoughts or feelings.

When you feel worthy, you will no longer feel a compulsion to constantly do something; you'll be comfortable just being.

So, let's start this chapter off with an easy questionnaire to determine if you are actually worth self-love and help from others. Check all of the boxes that apply.

- · I have murdered someone in cold blood.
- · I have raped someone.
- · I feel joy and fulfillment when I hurt someone else.

Pretty awful questions, aren't they? Did you check any of the boxes? I didn't think so...which means you are worth it. You are perfectly imperfect like every other person on earth, which means you are worth respect, love, and care. I can totally understand why you would hate yourself if you had murdered, raped or intentionally hurt someone, but short of those atrocities, why hate yourself for simply being imperfect? Have you hurt someone else? Probably. But those other people have hurt people too. Have you made mistakes? Most definitely, but so has everyone else. Have you had moments of laziness, selfishness, moodiness, failure, or weakness? Yeah, me too! Is your spouse/partner perfect? No. Are your kids perfect (try to be objective on this one)? No. Are your friends and family perfect? No and no. No one is perfect, and yet you think everyone else is worthy but you. Why?

As emotional eaters, one of the things we do is put ourselves in the position of martyr and take care of everyone else to the point of exhaustion with no energy left to take care of ourselves. And by taking on more than your share of the responsibilities at home, or using your own precious time, energy and money to solve other people's problems, or ignoring your needs to take care of your family, you are telling everyone around you that you are unworthy of being anyone's priority, including your own. Then we feel sorry for ourselves, and we feel resentful. So, we eat because we feel neglected, unloved and rundown. The simple truth is that we are doing that to ourselves. It's no one else's fault.

Instead of empowering others in your life with the ability to take care of themselves and their own problems, you are enabling them to become dependent on you so that, 1, you feel worthy of their love, and 2, so you don't have to focus on yourself. Let's work on those in order.

First of all, I want you to read the next statement out loud. "My worth has nothing to do with what I do for others, but with who I am." Say it again. Now, one more time.

What does this statement really mean?

What is your reaction to it?

Understanding and embracing that you are worthy of love, acceptance, care, protection, attention, loyalty, laughter, devotion and a large number of other things simply by **being** and not by **doing** is important. I want you to think about and write out all of the reasons why you are worthy, without writing down a single thing that you *do* for others.

For example, here is my list

I am positive, at least when I'm not hormonal	I love life...for the most part ☺
I am loyal to those that deserve it (not so much to those that don't ☺)	I am impatient but try to be otherwise (rarely successfully when I'm driving)
I am attentive... when I'm not busy being selfish... I'm the youngest child, so you know...	I have an open mind... most of the time
I love adventure, unless I'm feeling lazy	I love to laugh and see others laugh
I am accepting of others	I have a kind heart
I love to smile... when I'm not stressed out	I am assertive... unless I'm avoiding conflict
I gain pleasure from helping others	I am a leader
I am honest to a fault	I am decisive... unless I don't have the energy for it

I made myself laugh when I made this list. I am so obviously perfectly imperfect! ☺ And yet I am just as worthy of love as the people in my life who I love. *And so are you.*

So, take a few minutes and describe who you are and why you are worthy. Remember, don't list a single thing that you do.

Now look back on this list, reread it, and say, "This is who I am, and who I am is perfectly imperfect and worthy of love." This brings us back to my favorite quote from Eleanor Roosevelt. "No one can make you feel inferior without your consent." It is a great reminder that **WE** are the only ones who can make ourselves feel inferior. No one else is able to do that unless we allow it. So, the inverse is also true. No one can make us feel worthy unless we allow it; **YOU** are the only one who can make you feel worthy. The list above, no matter what you put on it, makes you worthy of love.

Are you still struggling to accept that? If so, you are probably a "do-er" that needs distractions to avoid looking too closely at yourself and your own problems and imperfections—just like me.

I always believed that if I just worked harder, thought smarter or acted kinder, I could be as close to perfect as possible. And it always pissed me off that I was never able to achieve perfection.

You know what's funny, or actually really sad, is that I spent so much of my life trying to be perfect only to learn that instead of being perfect, I was simply really boring. In an effort to be the "perfect" daughter, I never snuck out, I never broke curfew, I never dabbled with drugs, alcohol or sex, I didn't date, I rarely acted disrespectful or lied, and I never rebelled. As the "perfect" student I followed the dress code, raised my hand in class, got straight A's, handed in all of my assignments on time, participated in class, and was generally considered the teacher's pet because they all loved me, because I was so damn perfect. But you know what? All I got for all of that effort was approval from the authority figures in my life and derision from the other kids. It didn't win me any friends; it didn't lead to any great memories; it didn't create any great stories to share, it didn't win me any great life experiences. It didn't win me anything except maybe approval from the adults in my life. But, even then, I never approved of myself. No matter how "perfect" I was, I was never good enough.

Now, when friends and I reminisce about the good old days, I don't have anything to talk about. They, on the other hand, share stories and laughter about the various stunts they pulled as kids. They talk about the various fun or scary situations they experienced growing up. I don't really have any of those stories. I was too busy trying to be perfect to really live my life. Living means putting ourselves in a position of making mistakes. Making mistakes means you aren't perfect. If you aren't perfect, you aren't worth love, attention, respect or care. Right? Wrong! Wrong! Wrong!

Perfection is a bid for approval; it is externally focused, which inherently leads to failure. It is also a form of isolation that protects us from rejection. Perfect people are untouchable; they either intimidate others or make others feel uncomfortable because they feel like we are judging them for their own imperfections. It is a great way to isolate ourselves from any chance of being hurt by standing alone on the pedestal of perfection rather than diving into life and making mistakes that others can see.

But as you stand alone on that pedestal, you have nothing else to do but continue to judge yourself on your level of perfection, which ironically will never be absolutely perfect. You are perpetuating a cycle of self-disgust that will never allow you to feel any self-worth. So, instead, you keep yourself busy and distracted, focusing on everyone else's problems and needs so you don't have to look too closely at your own. Unfortunately, that just tends to exhaust you because your own problems are weighing heavily on your subconscious mind while everyone else's problems are weighing heavily on your conscious mind. This leads you to feeling rundown, taken advantage of and neglected, which compels you to emotionally eat.

So instead of taking care of everyone else's problems, let's try to feel worthy instead.

I think now is a good time to do a little dreaming. Imagine what your life would be like if your wants and needs were your greatest priority.

Seriously, I want you to put this book down for at least 5 or 10 minutes...hell, an hour, or however long you need! Close your eyes and visualize what your life would be like if you were a priority. Start with what you would do differently when you woke up in the morning and then take it from there.

Don't worry, I'll wait. Take your time.

I mean it! Shut this book right now, and go dream!

Welcome back! Now, I want you to write down what you saw in your dream. What did you see, experience, feel, and do in your dream?

What stops you from living that dream in reality?

| |
| |
| |
| |
| |
| |
| |
| |
| |

There's really only one word that you needed to write in response to that last question. Are you ready for the cold, hard truth? The answer is…YOU. You are the only one stopping yourself from being a priority. You may have kids, or a spouse/partner, family members, a demanding job, or other responsibilities that require your time and attention, but that doesn't mean your needs cannot be a priority too. You are worth it. You are worth just as much care and attention as everyone else you take care of. You are worth being taken care of. You are worth being cared for. You are worth being at the top of your priority list.

So, what does that mean? It means waking up each morning and thinking about what *you* need to have a happy, healthy day. Does that mean you need time to journal? Does that mean you need time to plan meals? Does that mean you need time to cook? Does that mean you need time to exercise? Does that mean you need time to meditate or sit in simple quietness? Does it mean you need time for a nap, a massage, a day without doing any cleaning?

Do you need to soak in a bathtub for twenty minutes and enjoy some peace and quiet, or some favorite music playing? Do you need to go for coffee with a friend? It's up to you. You are worth any one or all of those things, and more...even all at once! The more you give in to your needs and wants, the better you will feel, the happier you will become, and the better you will be for everyone else.

Women make better wives, mothers, friends, workers and daughters when they are happy and fulfilled. It is the same for men. And you can't be happy if you aren't taking care of yourself, if you aren't ensuring that your needs are met, if you aren't acting as if you are just as important as everyone else in your life.

If you are a parent, you know that your kids are sponges that mimic what they see. Is that how you want your kids to act as adults? Do you want them thinking that they are only worthy if they put everyone else's needs above their own? Because that is what you are teaching them when you don't take care of yourself or meet your own needs. And the simple fact is, your children are much more capable than you give them credit for. In fact, I want you to do a little experiment. The next time your child asks you to do something or to find something for them, don't do it. They may whine and they may cry, but if you stay firm, I will bet you a million dollars that they figure it out for themselves. I would then do that same experiment with your spouse, your co-workers, your friends and your family members. You will be shocked by how capable everyone else is when you stop doing everything for them. They may be resistant since you've trained them to rely on you, but if you can stay strong in the face of their resistance, all of you will get a great lesson. That lesson is that people, whether they are children, elderly or any age in between, are extremely capable when given the opportunity to be so.

With that in mind, what things are you currently doing for others that you should stop doing in order to create more time to take care of yourself?

| |
| |
| |
| |
| |
| |
| |
| |

What things from your dream list can you make a reality starting today or tomorrow?

| |
| |
| |
| |
| |
| |
| |
| |

Of everything on your dream list, what are the top three things that would make you feel loved and worthy each day?

| |
| |
| |
| |
| |
| |
| |

There is no time like the present to implement these changes. I want you to do at least one thing every single day to show yourself love. Then, as you get more comfortable with the idea, implement more and more changes into your daily life so that you constantly feel love for yourself. Once you begin to embrace the idea of loving yourself, you will be able to feel and accept love from others, which will help to fill the emotional gaps that compel you to reach for food.

CHAPTER 15

Focus Outward—Charity

As important as it is to start focusing on your wants and needs in a positive way, it is equally important to focus on *others* in a positive way. Emotional eaters tend to be hyper-critical and very self-focused. We are constantly assessing whether we have been perfect today. Have we done enough today? Are we worthy of love today? We are constantly beating ourselves up for doing this or saying that, eating this or drinking that. This level of self-focus is unhealthy. It is opposite to the kind of self-care I advocated in the last chapter.

A great way to get outside of yourself and start appreciating who you are and the life that you have is to live a life of gratitude. The easiest way to live a life of gratitude is to help others less fortunate than you; not out of obligation, not out of responsibility, but to create a sense of fulfillment and to recognize that you are a good person with a good life and you can do a lot of good in the world by loving yourself and sharing that love with others. I don't recommend volunteering for just any charity. Hell, you don't need to volunteer for a charity at all! Simply look for fulfilling opportunities to help others, opportunities that allow you to see the world with new, grateful eyes. Your help doesn't even need to be focused on humans. Volunteer to help animals, if that fulfills you! Dedicate time to pick up litter in your neighborhood or volunteer to start a recycling program at your office...whatever! Just find something that allows you to use your time and talents to help the world, opportunities to help those that truly need it; not those that simply rely on you because you let them.

Just to make sure we are on the same page, answer the following question.

Why did I advocate setting boundaries with friends and family in the last chapter just to encourage you to help others in this chapter? What is the difference?

The answer is simple: one drains you and one fulfills you. Allowing friends and family to take advantage of you in order to feel worthy is draining and demoralizing. Following a passion to help others and make the world a better place is fulfilling and will increase your self-confidence. Although the objective of helping people is the same, the underlying reason for doing it is completely different.

I want you to step outside of yourself and look at all of the good you can bring to the world. I want you to step outside of yourself and find opportunities to feel good about who you are and what you contribute. I want you to find opportunities to praise yourself for doing a great job at something besides overcoming your emotional eating, as important as that is. Your relationship with food has been a primary focal point in your life, and with that comes stress, depression, anxiety, and a constant state of hyper-awareness of your every thought, action and deed. It is time to focus your energy elsewhere, on something more positive and uplifting.

What activities to help others or to make the world a better place would give you a sense of satisfaction, pride and gratitude? (If you are drawing a blank, search Google and see what charities and organizations are in your area!)

| |
| |
| |
| |
| |
| |
| |

Let's double check that your heart is in the right place with the answers to the last question.

Look at each of the activities on your checklist and answer the following questions:

| Why will this activity bring me fulfillment? |
| Who or what am I helping, and do they really need it? Why? |

Awesome! You now have a great idea of what you can do to bring yourself a sense of pride and fulfillment while helping others. Isn't that fantastic?!

It will only remain fantastic if you do these activities from the right head and heart space, so, remind yourself that:

- There is no obligation to do any of these activities! You only do them when you want to do them.
- You don't have to do all of the activities at the same time. You can change your mind about which activities you participate in; maybe one year you'll do one, and the next year change to something else. You have choices!
- You don't have to dedicate hours, days, weeks, or months of your life to any of these activities. You have your own life to live. Only offer the amount of time you have to spare for that activity. In the same vein, don't rationalize your way out of doing it if you truly can fit it in. Do not use this as a reason to berate and punish yourself!

Now, let's focus on the logistics to ensure these activities actually come to life.

Do you have any idea where to take part in these activities? If not, then go do a Google search and find out.

Do you have a clear idea of how often you want to participate in these activities?

Thinking about your schedule, when is it most realistic that you will have the time and energy for these activities?

What will you do if one day you are too exhausted or too busy to complete the activity?

That last one was a trick question. I hope you wrote something like, "I will take care of myself first and wait until a better time to help the world." You know how on airplanes the stewards/stewardesses always tell you to put the face mask on yourself FIRST, and then help the child or person next to you? The same principle applies here. You must help yourself first in order to be able to help others. If you don't feel up to volunteering on the day you had planned, feel really good about rescheduling in order to keep yourself healthy in mind, body and spirit. That is what this entire journey is about— creating a head and heart space, as well as a life, that allows your mental, spiritual, and physical state to be at its peak. Love yourself first. Help yourself first. Heal yourself first. Then, find opportunities to share your love, help and healing with others.

CHAPTER 16

Summary

Whew! You did it! You've diligently worked through the various activities in this book to work towards better balance and peace with yourself and with food; you've learned how to *Feel Not Food*.

How do you feel?

Although the activities themselves may have been draining, if you took your time to work through the process, then by now you should feel lighter and freer! That sense of lightness comes from finally understanding the root cause of your emotional eating challenges and knowing that you now have tools to help you overcome them. That sense of being free comes from no longer feeling that you are controlled by food or your own self-sabotaging thoughts.

Doesn't it feel good? Hold that feeling in your heart and embrace it! Embrace that feeling of self-satisfaction, peace, freedom, relief, excitement, and any other feelings you may be experiencing as a result of completing your transformation. This is a time for celebration and pride! Not because you are "healed," not because you are no longer an emotional eater, not because food no longer controls you, but because you now understand the truth behind your behaviors and challenges. And with that understanding comes freedom.

You now understand many things, including

1. that there is no "cure" for emotional eating. There are simply techniques you can employ on your life-long journey to reduce the tendency to emotionally eat, so you can live a healthier, happier life.
2. that weight is not your problem, so you can stop hyper-focusing on it. Simply eat mindfully with the objective of being healthy and your weight will fall in line.
3. what changes you are and are not willing to make on this journey. You also understand that your willingness to change will evolve, as well. Focusing on easy wins creates a pleasant journey filled with feelings of success rather than failure. Your ability to handle more difficult changes comes with the feelings of success you experience when you adopt changes that are easier to make.

4. being self-aware is crucial to success, so consistently keeping journals for both your food and your emotions can help to keep you honest and in touch with yourself.
5. in order to truly live, you must allow yourself to feel. The reality is that if you squelch one emotion you squelch them all, so that even positive emotions like love and happiness can't be felt to their fullest capacity if you squelch emotions like anger and sadness.
6. food is neither good nor bad, it is simply nourishment for our bodies. By creating other avenues for rewards, celebrations, distraction, and comfort you don't have to rely on food to bring you fulfillment in these situations.
7. you are perfectly imperfect; therefore, you deserve self-compassion when you aren't at your best. It is important to keep yourself accountable, but accountability should always be balanced with self-compassion.
8. to build self-confidence, you have to recognize and acknowledge when you have done things well. Every small success matters and you should acknowledge it. Say your "praise phrase" often!
9. life is not black and white. You now understand the importance of keeping your attitudes and thoughts in perspective. You now understand the importance of taking judgment and emotion out of things that don't deserve it. Feel comfortable living in the gray.
10. triggers come in many forms such as foods, emotions and circumstances. You should now have a plan for either avoiding them or dealing with them.
11. stress is a big contributor to emotional eating. Being honest about what really needs to be on your plate and what can be taken off will help you from feeling overwhelmed and turning to food for energy and comfort.
12. who is part of your support system and what you need from them. Success is always easier with support.

13. that you deserve to be taken care of—by yourself and by others. You are just as important as everyone else in your life, therefore you must make yourself a priority so others will, too. You deserve it.
14. living a life of gratitude will help you to appreciate who you are and the life you lead. By spending your valuable time volunteering to help those less fortunate than yourself, you get out of your head, build your self-worth, increase feelings of pride and begin experiencing your life with gratitude rather than resentment.

You have learned so much as you worked through the various activities in this book!

The key is to continue to use the knowledge and techniques you have gained through this process; transformation is a continual evolution that doesn't end with the completion of this book. Consider this book as a catalyst for continued growth and learning so that you never revert back to old, self-sabotaging habits. Instead, continue to work through the various activities in this book as you need them to help you remain successful on this journey. Continued success fosters pride and self-confidence, which will help you embrace who you are and the value you bring to the world.

And when you experience moments of failure, as we all do, show yourself compassion and remember you are perfectly imperfect and are worthy of love and forgiveness. Then pick yourself back up, recognize that you are both capable and worthy of being successful, and get back on track. Build your self-confidence, so you feel capable of taking on any challenge despite any fear or setback you may experience. Look in the mirror with pride, because you are actively overcoming one of your greatest challenges. Then get out there and live your healthiest, most fulfilling life!

You deserve it!

ADDITIONAL RESOURCES

Books that Inspire and Teach You to Create an Amazing Life

The Four Agreements: A Practical Guide to Personal Freedom – Don Miguel Ruiz

Be Amazing: Tools for Living Inspired – Erin Ramsey

You Are A Badass: How to Stop Doubting Your Greatness and Start Living an Awesome Life – Jen Sincero

E^2: Nine Do It Yourself Energy Experiments That Prove Your Thoughts Create Reality – Pam Grout

Ask and It Is Given: Learning to Manifest Your Desires – Esther and Jerry Hicks

Books that Teach You to Accept and Love Yourself as You Are, and Create Stronger Connections with Others

The Power of Vulnerability - Brené Brown (a favorite author – all of her books are great and I recommend watching her TED Talks)

The Gifts of Imperfection - Brené Brown

Daring Greatly - Brené Brown

Self Parenting: The Complete Guide to Your Inner Conversations: *Learn to Love, Support and Nurture Your "Inner" Child* - John K. Pollard, III

Books that Teach You How to Eat for Healthy Body

The Hunger Fix - Dr. Pamela Peeke

The Eat Clean Diet - Tosca Reno

Made in the USA
San Bernardino, CA
06 March 2020